Selecting and Using Breastfeeding Tools

Improving Care and Outcomes

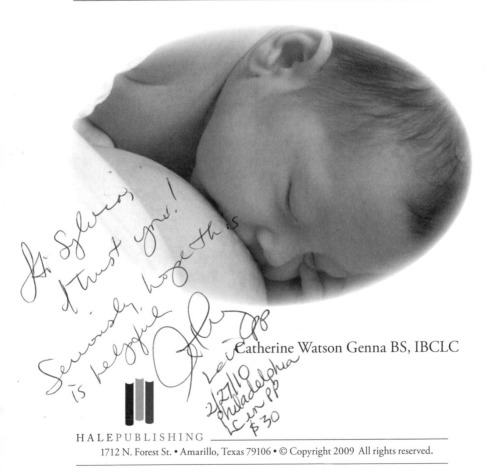

Catherine Watson Genna BS, IBCLC

HALEPUBLISHING
1712 N. Forest St. • Amarillo, Texas 79106 •

Selecting and Using Breastfeeding Tools
Improving Care and Outcomes

Catherine Watson Genna BS, IBCLC

© Copyright 2009

Hale Publishing, L.P.

1712 N. Forest St.

Amarillo, TX   79106-7017

806-376-9900

800-378-1317

www.iBreastfeeding.com

www.hale-publishing.com

Printed in Canada.

Library of Congress Control Number: 2009929774

ISBN-13: 978-0-9823379-1-2

Table of Contents

Dedication

This book is dedicated to those who built the knowledge and skills that our profession uses daily to assist breastfeeding families, and those who contributed to my personal skill set.

My grandfathers had a way with tools: Grandpa Watson was a machinist, and frequently designed or modified tools to solve problems. Grandpa Ferrara was a printer, and was the go-to guy when a machine balked, jammed or stalled. Dad built beauty on large and small scales, enlarging and repairing our house, and later making lovely furniture, often with Mom at his side. I thank them all for the legacy of both nature and nurture.

I am indebted to the colleagues who provided the backbone of our practice. Though their names may no longer be attached to their ideas and innovations, many dyads have benefited. I am grateful to those who generously contributed to this book. No one of us can know everything, but with our constant sharing and examination of new and old ideas, we can continue to build a body of tools and techniques to help families to breastfeed.

May we continue to learn together, and perhaps more importantly, to un-learn that which Mark Twain identified as the "trouble with the world," that we "know so many things that just aren't so."

- Catherine Watson Genna

Introduction

Ideally, breastfeeding is initiated within minutes after birth, is comfortable and effective for both mother and infant, and remains so until the child outgrows the need for both human milk and the autonomic regulation derived from breastfeeding. Unfortunately, breastfeeding is a complex system, and every biological system sometimes breaks down. Breastfeeding was already in decline when birth moved into hospitals in the 1930s. Birth procedures and routines developed before the physiology of lactation and mechanics of breastfeeding were understood, allowing interventions (labor analgesia and anesthesia, maternal-infant separation, and supplemental feeding) which interfere with breastfeeding to become entrenched. In addition, medical technology is now able to save babies with a low likelihood of survival without skilled care. These infants often have significant feeding problems related to anatomical, neurological, or cardiorespiratory lesions, or immaturity. These are some of the reasons there is a need for skilled lactation assistance and tools to support or enhance breastfeeding in problematic situations.

Research into the science of breastfeeding and human lactation is teaching us how lactation and breastfeeding work. Science has provided a basis for practice, but every nuance of how to help individual mothers is not covered by existing randomized controlled trials. When we reach the end of what is demonstrated by research, we cautiously rely on the pattern recognition skills of the human brain, with the realization that sometimes the patterns are imposed rather than real. Expert opinion is based on long experience with different nuances within a specialty practice and is looked to when there is no stronger evidence. Case series provide evidence for clinical patterns. Uncontrolled trials help refine treatments and procedures, but are not as reliable as studies containing a control group. Randomized controlled trials (RCTs) compare two or more treatments. When well designed and executed, RCTs can provide valuable information to guide practice. However, some studies (particularly industry sponsored ones) "stack the deck" in favor of the manufacturer's product in their design, or suffer from shoddy analysis or over-application of the findings. For example, a study comparing a manual breast pump to a small, single consumer grade electric pump already on the market was touted as demonstrating that the manual pump was superior to electric breast pumps. This monograph will describe tools that can be helpful in lactation consultant practice, critically review the existing research on each tool category, and then provide clinical guidance for effective use of each individual tool.

Why Use Tools?

Why would we need to use tools? While it is ideal to keep mothers and babies together and breastfeeding, and manual expression of milk can work very well when they need to be separated; a technological society has come up with devices that can reduce the work involved in maintaining milk production or feeding a baby who is not yet able to breastfeed without intervention. Breastfeeding problems involve two persons and their interactions, making randomized trials of interventions difficult to conduct. Moreover, breastfeeding is a robust process and usually requires multiple "hits" before it becomes unworkable, so many dyads seen in private practice have more than one issue.

In a lactation consultation, clinical reasoning guides our choice of interventions. Clinical reasoning requires a firm background in the science, including the sociology and psychology, of breastfeeding. What we observe and intuit about the dyad informs our choice of interventions to make breastfeeding work for that family. Assessment and observation may reveal that a complex tool is ideal for a dyad's breastfeeding problem, but intuition (the natural ability of the brain to make accurate judgments based on subtle and often incomplete information) may point out the mother's emotional fragility and lead to the choice of an easier to use, though less efficient intervention.

The first rule of lactation is "feed the baby," but breastfeeding is so much more than the provision of nutrition. Trophic compounds direct the development of the infant's commensal gut flora, the immune system, the lining of the intestines, and the brain. The process of suckling properly develops facial musculature and bones, such that children who were bottle fed have a greater risk of malocclusion (Carrascoza et al., 2006; Lescano de & Varela, 2006), which is compounded by the more frequent use of pacifiers in bottle fed children (Leite-Cavalcanti et al., 2007). Studies have found that bottle fed children have poorer voice tonal quality (Broad, 1975) and, in boys, a strong deficit in speech articulation clarity (Broad & Duganzich, 1983).

Brian Palmer, DDS, first noticed that his breastfed patients had a wider palate and better dental health than his bottle fed ones. He verified this observation by examining prehistoric versus modern jaws and teeth. Dr. Palmer believes a wide palate contributes to normal breathing during sleep by widening the nasopharynx and posterior nasal apertures (Palmer, 1998). He has demonstrated through specialized photography that normal tongue function, normal palate width, and wider choanae (the passageways from the back of each side of the nose to the throat) are associated with the presence of breastfeeding and the absence of tongue-tie.

The normal aerobic exercise of breastfeeding influences lung development in infants. Lung volume and airflow (FEV) has been found to be reduced in children who were not breastfed (Ogbuanu et al., 2009). It has long been postulated that there is crosstalk between the baby's saliva and the mother's immune system during breastfeeding. Just recently, researchers have demonstrated that cells from the baby's saliva do enter the breast (Densmore & Pflueger, 2008). The sensory and psychological importance of breastfeeding is harder to measure. In all, direct breastfeeding is well worth working toward.

Choosing Tools

The goal of tool use is to help dyads to breastfeed who are otherwise unable to do so. Therefore, tools and techniques that make direct breastfeeding possible or more effective are more desirable than those that separate mom and baby. There are certainly times when the infant is unable to breastfeed even with tools, and alternate feeding and milk removal methods are needed while the infant gains or regains the ability to feed normally. A wise choice of alternate feeding methods can help the infant develop the feeding skills that are necessary for direct breastfeeding. Sometimes maternal issues, such as significant nipple damage, result in the need for tools. Again, preserving at-breast feeding is primary. Therefore, tools will be covered in order of their preservation of direct breastfeeding.

Sore Nipple Treatments

Nipple pain is a common complaint of women seeking lactation assistance, and many products are sold to treat it. While finding and addressing the cause of sore nipples is always the primary concern, there is a high demand for creams, gels, and dressings that reduce pain or improve healing. Most studies of sore nipple treatments involve small samples and compare only two or three treatments, making it difficult to identify particularly effective ones within the breastfeeding literature. In this section, products for treating sore nipples are discussed, drawing upon research from other fields as needed.

Moist Wound Healing

Moist wound healing is the control of moisture in a wound to speed skin repair. In full thickness wounds (those in which all skin structures are destroyed), the correct moisture balance preserves the ability of skin cells, specifically keratinocytes, to detach from the wound edges and migrate along the framework laid down by platelets during clotting (Falanga & Iwamoto, 2008). The large body of research on moist wound healing provides information applicable to injured nipple care (Cable et al., 1997).

> *"Based on current knowledge of the cascade of biochemical and cellular events involved in wound healing, clinicians have come to accept and understand that use of dry dressings retards healing" (Eisenbud et al., 2003).*

Moist wound healing can be accomplished with different materials. Hydrogels, modified lanolins, and medical (radiation-sterilized) honey are all moist wound healing methods that can be used on nipple wounds. The important factor is to maintain proper tissue moisture balance to prevent scabbing from dehydration or maceration from over hydration. Dressings that promote moist wound healing increase the speed of healing by maintaining the fluid environment tissue-building chemicals need to function, increase the action of cells and enzymes that painlessly break down and remove dead tissue (autolytic debridement), and significantly reduce pain. The mechanism of this pain relief is unknown, but it may be at least partially due to covering exposed nerve endings.

Hydrogels

Hydrogels, dressings made of a water gel in a supportive polymer framework, come in many formulations. Polymers with various degrees of cross-linking lead to different levels of firmness of the gel, and different polymer side chains (the part of the hydrogel that attracts water) help determine absorbency. Very soft gels may be better at conforming to the wound surface and relieving pain, but may need to have another dressing (secondary dressing) placed over them. Firmer gels provide better protection from friction of movement against clothing. However, most hydrogel dressings are appropriate for most nipple wounds, and differences between products are fairly minor. Allergies and extremes of leakage (which might destroy the integrity of less absorbent dressings) would be reasons to change to a different formulation. Otherwise, convenience, ability of the form factor to fill the wound and relieve pain, and cost per day of use can guide choice of brands.

Hydrogel pads or sheets are designed for relatively shallow wounds. They may soften as they absorb wound fluids, improving their ability to reach into the nooks and crannies of the wound. Amorphous (unformed) hydrogel comes in tubes or similar dispensers and is spread on the wound with a specially designed applicator or with a scrupulously clean finger or sterile swab. Amorphous hydrogel is able to penetrate into deeper wounds. Because it has no backing, it is not occlusive, so it can potentially be used on infected tissue (on top of an antibiotic treatment). Amorphous hydrogel is able to "donate" more moisture to the wound than a sheet dressing can, though as a rule, hydrogels are able to donate or absorb moisture as required by the wound.

Since nipples secrete milk in addition to wound exudates (blood serum and intercellular fluids leaked by wounds), hydrogels used on the nipple area should be particularly absorbent or should allow a lot of moisture to travel from the nipple to the environment through their matrix and any backing material. Hydrogel backing sheets are typically semi-occlusive and permeable to oxygen, carbon dioxide, and other gases. The amount of water transmitted through the gel (including the backing sheet) is termed the moisture vapor transmission rate (MVTR). A hydrogel without a backing or with a high MVTR is likely a better choice for mothers who leak a lot of milk.

Hydrogels can also be formulated with additives that change their properties. Natural substances derived from seaweed (alginates) can increase absorbency of a dressing and autolytic debridement (Okan et al., 2007). Alginates help control bleeding (improve hemostasis). Alginates should be rinsed off the breast with warm water before breastfeeding to avoid infant ingestion, though there are no known harmful effects of the ingredients. An example of an alginate-containing hydrogel that is appropriate for use on nipples is ConvaTec SafGel.

Saline hydrogels can increase autolytic debridement and should not have adverse effects on nipples. Again, the nipple area should be rinsed to avoid infant ingestion of any traces on the breast. Other dressing additives include silver particles and other antimicrobials designed to be released into the wound. Researchers are experimenting with dressings that affect growth factors and absorb or inactivate bacterial products that interfere with healing. Currently, no research has been done on the use of antimicrobial or bioactive additives on lactating nipples or their safety for breastfeeding infants.

Hydrogels differ in composition and should be used according to their manufacturer's directions. Some are designed to be rinsed (e.g., Ameda Comfort Gel Pads and Medela Tender Care Hydrogels), and others are not (e.g., Soothies). Rinsing hydrogels that are not designed for contact with water can cause them to disintegrate or become oversaturated, which increases the risk of wound maceration. Some hydrogels have a stiffer polymer matrix and are made to be used without a covering; others are formulated to allow excess water to evaporate, despite having a cloth or perforated plastic backing. Absorption and moisture vapor transmission characteristics determine how long an individual hydrogel dressing can be used.

Contraindications

Infection

Occlusive or semi-occlusive dressings like hydrogel sheets or pads are not recommended for use on infected tissue (Cable et al., 1997; Cable & Davis, 1998). When nipple skin is broken, hygiene is important to prevent mastitis from ascending bacteria (Livingstone & Stringer, 1999). Washing injured nipples twice daily with mild soap and water can reduce the number of bacteria present and reduce the risk of mastitis. The surrounding tissue is the most frequent source of microorganisms that infect wounds. Infected nipples require medical treatment (Porter & Schach, 2004) to prevent the organisms from moving up the ductal tree.

Brent et al. (1998) set out to study the use of hydrogels on sore nipples compared to the established treatment of medical grade modified lanolin cream and breast shells used together after allowing expressed milk to air-dry on the nipples. Only women without signs of nipple infection were accepted into the study, and all mothers received positioning and latch assistance. The researchers discontinued the study when 7 of 21 patients in the hydrogel group developed infections and one patient developed dermatitis compared with 2 infections in the lanolin group. The Elasto-gel dressings (the direct predecessor of Soothies) in this study were changed at every feeding. It is possible that the frequent changes of dressing increased the risk of infection. Soothies are a relatively tacky hydrogel of those marketed for use on lactating breasts, and they are stickiest when they are new. It is possible that using a new dressing at each feeding interfered with healing. In this study, there was a non-significant trend toward better healing in the lanolin group.

The increased incidence of mastitis reported by Brent et al. was not found in studies of other hydrogel dressings (Benbow & Vardy-White, 2004). In fact, in a study randomizing postpartum women to prophylactic use of either modified lanolin (Lansinoh) application after expressing milk onto their nipples versus rinsing the breast and applying hydrogels (MaterniMates), there were no infections in the hydrogel group and seven infections in the lanolin group (Dodd & Chalmers, 2003). Rinsing the baby's oral secretions off the breast before using the hydrogels and rinsing the breast after removing the gels before breastfeeding may have been responsible for the absence of infection. MaterniMates are now distributed in the U.S. as Ameda Comfort Gels by Ameda Breastfeeding Products. Ameda recommends rinsing the breasts before and after hydrogel use. Other manufacturers also recommend rinsing the breast before applying their hydrogels and after removing them to breastfeed, including Medela, Maternal Concepts, and Hygeia. This is good advice and should be reinforced with clients.

HELPFUL TIPS

IF A DRESSING IS DIFFICULT OR PAINFUL TO REMOVE, FLOOD IT WITH CLEAN WATER OR STERILE SALINE UNTIL IT RELEASES FROM THE WOUND. THIS GENERALLY DESTROYS THE DRESSING, BUT PRESERVES THE HEALING PROGRESS.

A recent review of the literature showed that hydrogel dressings neither promote infection nor provide superior protection against infection as compared to traditional dry dressings (Slater, 2008). My own clinical experience with hydrogels has been positive, as I stress washing injured nipples with mild soap and water twice daily. Hydrogels are a very gratifying product to provide to mothers, who almost invariably sigh with relief upon application.

Allergic Reactions

Rarely, an allergic reaction to a constituent of a hydrogel may occur, consisting of a red rash in the area covered by the dressing. Figure 1 shows a typical allergic rash to a hydrogel pad. The red raised rash covers the entire area exposed to the pad. Allergic reactions tend to continue to worsen with repeated or prolonged exposure to an allergen. If an allergic rash occurs, the product should be immediately discontinued and the area washed with mild soap and water to remove any residue.

If an allergic reaction occurs to a hydrogel, a hydrogel with a different polymer, a medical honey, or modified lanolin can be substituted, or nipple treatments can be discontinued. If the rash fails to resolve promptly, the mother's healthcare practitioner may prescribe the use of a topical corticosteroid (hydrocortisone) cream. If a steroid is recommended, a very small amount (such that that the cream is not visible after application) should be applied with clean hands immediately after breastfeeding. Topical medications are meant to be absorbed by the skin, so rinsing before breastfeeding is usually not necessary unless a large amount is used. Hydrocortisone ointment (0.5-1%) is rated L2 by Dr. Hale (Hale, 2008) when used in small quantities, as transfer into milk is believed to be minimal. Hydrocortisone ointment or cream should be used for short periods of time (up to 10 days) to avoid thinning of the skin.

Figure 1. Allergic reaction to hydrogel

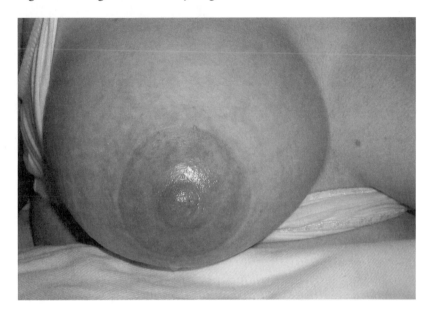

Raynaud's Syndrome or Vasospasm

Mothers should be screened for vasospasm before being offered hydrogel or glycerin gel dressings. Vasospasm is a reflex constriction of blood vessels in the skin, reducing blood supply and usually causing pain. Figure 2 shows the blanching that accompanies nipple vasospasm. Hydrogel and glycerin gel dressings allow moisture to move toward and away from the nipple. The cooling sensation mothers report is caused by evaporation of water from the nipple surface, which takes heat (energy) from the body. Evaporative cooling may be problematic in mothers with vasospasm, as chilling is a trigger for this condition, though individual sensitivity to the amount of moisture movement with hydrogels will vary. Mothers with vasospasm who do not tolerate hydrogels can be advised to immediately pat their nipples dry to avoid evaporative chilling, and then cover them with something that preserves warmth, such as a wool nursing pad. Wool wicks excess moisture away from the nipple, allowing it to evaporate from the surface of the wool rather than from the skin. Untreated wool nursing pads are sold by Danish Woolen Delight Danish Woolen Delight (LANACare Nursing Pads - www.danishwool.com) and Maternal Concepts (SofteN Nursing Pads - www.maternalconcepts.com).

HELPFUL TIPS

WHEN USING A HYDROGEL DRESSING, MAKE SURE THE DRESSING COVERS THE ENTIRE WOUND PLUS A MARGIN OF AT LEAST A FEW MILLIMETERS AROUND THE EDGES OF THE WOUND. KEEPING THE WOUND EDGES MOIST ALLOWS CELLS (KERATINOCYTES) TO DETACH FROM THE EDGES AND MIGRATE INTO THE INTERIOR OF THE WOUND TO PRODUCE NEW TISSUE. MOTHERS OFTEN CUT HYDROGELS TO SAVE MONEY. INSTRUCTING THEM ON HOW MUCH AREA NEEDS TO BE COVERED ALLOWS THEM TO CUT TO THE PROPER SIZE.

Figure 2. Nipple Vasospasm

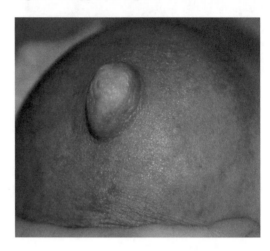

Hydrogel Products in Common Use for Nipple Healing

Amorphous Hydrogels

Derma Sciences AquaSite

Derma Sciences AquaSite amorphous hydrogel is a carbomer 940 based gel containing sterile water and glycerin. It comes in a 1 ounce plastic bellows container for ease of application. The container's applicator helps avoid contamination. Amorphous hydrogels are particularly good for filling deep or jagged wounds.

Use

Clean the wound and squeeze the container to dispense sufficient hydrogel to fill the wound to the level of the surrounding tissue. Cover with another dressing, such as a gauze pad or a clean nursing pad.

Price

The wholesale price for a case of 12 containers is around $40.

Contact Information

Derma Sciences www.dermasciences.com
1.800.445.7627

Advantages

- Very inexpensive per use
- Good for partial and full thickness wounds

Disadvantages

- Requires secondary dressing over the gel
- Not specifically tested on lactating nipples

Suggested Uses

- Deep or jagged wounds
- Mothers with poorer wound healing (rinsing does not disrupt healing tissue)

ConvaTec Saf-Gel

Figure 3. ConvaTec Saf-Gel

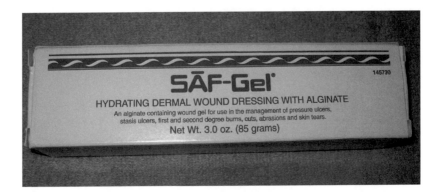

SafGel (figure 3) is an amorphous hydrogel with alginate for increased absorbency. Though some alginate dressings have a foul odor, SafGel has a barely detectable mild chemical odor. SafGel is completely water soluble and can be rinsed off the nipple with a stream of warm water before feeding. A tube is meant for single patient use (application with a dirty finger could theoretically contaminate the tube). If contact with the tube outlet is avoided, SafGel can be divided into multiple small sterile airtight containers (I use Snappies 13 ml colostrum containers) to safely give individual mothers smaller portions to avoid waste. Convatec has confirmed that SafGel remains active for 45 days after opening. No research has been done beyond 45 days. However, I've used SafGel that was opened for many months on my own full-thickness surgical wound with good results. SafeGel was not specifically tested on nipple skin, but the material safety data sheet shows there are no toxic ingredients.

Use

Wash hands with soap and water. Apply a 2mm deep film to the wound and 1-2 mm surrounding it, and cover with a secondary dressing (gauze or soft nursing pad). Rinse the breast with water before breastfeeding.

Price

About $14

Contact information

ConvaTec USA http://www.convatec.com

1.800.422.8811

Advantages

- Indicated for both partial and full thickness wounds
- Rinses off easily with water or saline
- Is particularly absorbent
- Keeps secondary dressing from sticking to the wound
- Contains only non-toxic ingredients

Disadvantages

- Requires secondary dressing
- Not specifically tested on lactating nipples, but all ingredients are non-toxic.

Suggested For

- Mothers with significant milk leakage
- Mothers whose infants breastfeed very often
- Mothers whose healing tissue is delicate and disrupted by removing a tackier hydrogel pad (it rinses off very easily without disrupting newly healing tissue)

Ameda Comfort Gel Pads

Figure 4. Ameda Comfort Gels

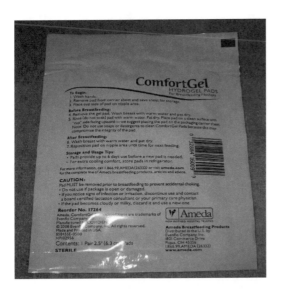

Ameda Comfort Gel Pads (figure 4) are a high density polyurethane based hydrogel formulation that is designed to be rinsed with warm water between uses to remove milk proteins and restore water that has evaporated from the pad. They were cleared by the FDA for use on shallow-to-full thickness wounds (Dodd & Chalmers, 2003). They are available in either sealed packets of one pair or retail packages containing two packets, providing a spare sterile pair. This product has no backing and a high moisture vapor transmission rate of 8300 g/m2/day, making them particularly effective for women with significant leakage of milk. The pads can be refrigerated between uses to enhance their cooling properties.

Use

The pads are gently contoured (like a contact lens) and will stay on better if placed with the concave side toward the breast. They should be rinsed and patted dry before re-use, and discarded when the clear hydrogels turn cloudy from absorbing milk proteins. They are designed to be used without other creams or ointments. Rinsing the baby's saliva off the breast after feeding and before replacing the gel pad may help prevent mastitis and is recommended by Ameda when using Comfort Gel Pads. Rinsing the breast before breastfeeding is also recommended.

Price

$10-12 per pair

Contact Information

Ameda Breastfeeding Products http://www.ameda.com

1.866.99.AMEDA

Advantages

- High density pad may protect from friction better than thinner pads.
- Can be used longer than other hydrogel products (4-6 days), decreasing per day cost.
- Can be rinsed to remove surface milk proteins.
- Developed specifically for use on lactating breasts, studied on lactating breasts
- Package includes a plastic liner that can be reused to keep the rinsed Comfort Gels clean during feeding.

Disadvantages

- More difficult to find, though availability is increasing.

Suggested Uses

- This product may be particularly helpful when nipples are painful to touch. Mothers have found the firmer matrix protected their nipples from friction from clothing.
- Good for mothers with significant milk leakage - high MVTR

Maternal Concepts Cooling Care Disposable Hydrogel Nursing Relief Pads

Figure 5. Maternal Concepts Cooling Care Pads

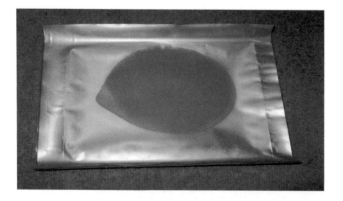

Cooling Care hydrogels (figure 5) are made from a non-toxic PEO (polyethylene oxide) based polymer and water, and are modeled on burn dressings. The package contains 12 soft dressings, packaged in 6 sterile pouches. Current package directions say they are for use on sore nipples, but not for use on cracked, bleeding, or blistered nipples, and that each pair should be used for no more than 30-60 minutes. However, the distributor's product specialist confirmed that they are safe for open wounds; they can be used for at least several hours at a time; and the package instructions are being revised.

Use

Maternal Concepts recommends that mothers wash their breasts and pat them dry before and after using Cooling Care dressings. The blue liner is removed and the gel side of the pad placed over the nipple area. The colorless liner is left in place to protect the integrity of the pad and maintain moisture balance, as well as to keep it from sticking to the bra.

Price

$12 per package of 12, discounts available for multiple box purchases

Contact Information

Maternal Concepts http://www.maternalconcepts.com/

1.800. 310.5817

Advantages

- Inexpensive
- Thin and soft - conforms well to breast (may be useful for narrower breasts)
- Teardrop shape provides a "handle" for holding dressing, potentially improving hygiene
- Frequent changing as recommended may reduce the risk of infection
- Strong cooling sensation due to high water movement

Disadvantages

- Soft dressing has lower integrity, strength, and absorbency. Leaving the colorless plastic backing on as instructed helps improve strength and integrity.
- May be less suitable for mothers with vasospasm

Suggested Use

- These dressings are particularly moist and non-adherent. They may better protect delicate newly-healing nipple wounds than tackier dressings. Since they are modeled on burn dressings, they are very helpful on breast burns as well.

Medela Tender Care Hydrogels

Figure 6. Medela Tender Care Hydrogels

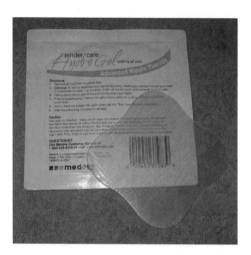

These thin hydrogels are made of water, glycerol, and a trade secret polymer with a semi-occlusive backing. They are sticky if not rinsed. The manufacturer's instructions recommend rinsing for 1-2 seconds twice a day, shaking to remove excess water, and then waiting 2 minutes before applying them. This allows the hydrogels to absorb a limited amount of water to reduce stickiness and increase surface smoothness for improved comfort. Water evaporates from these hydrogels at a faster rate in cold or dry climates, in which case they should be rinsed more often, up to five times a day. It is optimal to instruct mothers to rinse them when the pads feel less comfortable, between two and five times per day. The package recommends not rinsing more than twice a day, which a product specialist at Medela explained was chosen for the sake of simplicity and brevity. Lactation consultants (LCs) can help optimize use of this product by individualizing their instructions based on the local climate and weather.

Tender Care HydroGels are meant to be used for about 24 hours and then discarded. They should be discarded sooner if they become visibly white and opaque from milk absorption. When significant milk is absorbed by the pads, moisture content may approach levels that saturate the pad (95% water level), exposing the wound to potential maceration.

Use

Rinse pad briefly (1-2 seconds), shake off, allow to sit for two minutes before applying. Do this procedure 2-5 times a day according to environmental conditions (see above). Medela recommends washing the breast with warm water and patting dry both before application of the gel pads and before breastfeeding while using Tender Care Hydrogels.

Price

$13-15 for 4 pads (2 pairs) per box, a two day supply.

Contact Information

Medela, Inc. http://www.medelabreastfeedingus.com/

1.800.435.8316

Advantages

- Readily available in retail stores, mothers can buy them themselves
- Can be used over modified lanolins (helps keep lanolin from soiling bra and dressing from sticking to wound, but this increases costs)
- High moisture vapor transmission rate (but less absorbency than other products)
- Can be rinsed briefly to plump up gel and improve comfort
- Glycerol may provide bacteriostatic effect, but this specific formulation has not been tested.

Disadvantages

- Very tacky
- Difficult to remove if not used with lanolin, according to Kathleen Mirra, MEd, IBCLC (Flooding with saline or water will destroy dressing, but will cause it to release the healing tissue).
- Relatively expensive
- Relatively low absorbency, needs to be discarded faster if mother leaks more
- Some mothers report that the squared cloverleaf shape is more apparent through thin clothing than round hydrogels.

Suggested Uses

- General purpose moist wound healing dressing, best used over USP modified lanolin. Since Tender Care gels are individually wrapped, if only one pad is needed, the others will stay sterile.

Soothies

Figure 7. Soothies

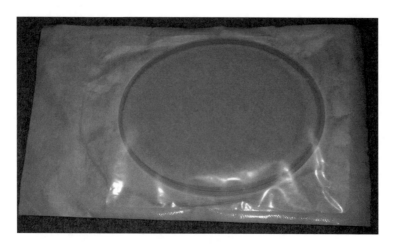

Soothies (figure 7) are made from a glycerin matrix. Glycerin has properties that stop the growth of microorganisms (i.e., is bacteriostatic) on contact. Only microorganisms that enter the gel pad are affected; the glycerin does not seem to migrate to the skin.

Soothies are meant to be used right from the package after removal of the plastic cover from the gel. The gel surface is placed against the nipple area; the cloth backing is left on and placed away from the skin. They are designed to be worn all the time except during bathing or showering, breastfeeding, or expressing milk. They can be refrigerated in an airtight plastic zipper-top bag (to prevent them from picking up moisture) between uses to enhance their cooling effect. They are very tacky and can injure skin if not removed carefully. They work best on mothers with moderate leakage of milk. Women with very low leakage rates or whose babies' breastfeed very frequently may find that they stick too well and may tear off healing tissues. Women with high leakage may have to discard them more often than the intended 24-48 hours.

Use

Soothies should be used without rinsing and should be discarded when the pad is no longer slightly tacky to the touch. They can be cut in half or quarters if the area needing coverage is small. The manufacturer recommends cutting the pads with the plastic cover in place with clean scissors to avoid contamination and reduce sticking to the scissors.

Price

$10-15 per pair

Contact Information

Soothies has been acquired by Lansinoh Laboratories http://www.lansinoh.com

1.800.292.4794

Advantages

- Provides significant pain relief
- Helps modulate moisture balance in shallow wounds to promote a moist wound healing environment
- Available in retail pharmacies

Disadvantages

- Tackiness can injure healing skin if not removed carefully (Flood with saline if they stick.)
- Expensive
- Usable for only 24-48 hours
- Increased infection rate in one study, not replicated in others

Suggested Use

- It's best to recommend Soothies for women with shallow (partial thickness) nipple injuries, moderate milk leakage, and no sign of infection. Signs of infection include purulence (creamy white or yellow discharge), golden crusting, or friable (easily broken) skin (figure 8). Advise washing the injured nipples with mild soap and water twice a day, and instruct mother to discontinue use if pain increases or signs of infection occur. Because Soothies are particularly tacky, they may stay in place better for mothers who do not wear a bra. If the dressing has only been worn a short time or the mother does not leak much, it may injure the granulation (healing) tissue if pulled off. Water or saline can be used to flood the dressing to loosen it safely.

Figure 8. Infected nipple

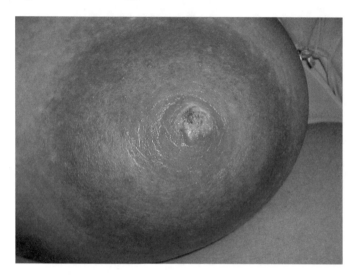

USP Modified Lanolin

Lanolin is a waxy substance produced by sheep's skin to coat their wool to protect it from the elements. Since it is similar in composition to human sebum, it is commonly used to lubricate skin and has long been an ingredient in nipple ointments. Lanolin is collected from wool after shearing and is washed off the wool by detergents. Unmodified lanolin can contain potentially toxic pesticides used on sheep ("sheep dip"), as well as allergenic detergent residues and free wool alcohols. The United States Pharmacopoeia (USP) requires medical grade lanolin to be purified to remove most of these substances. Products that meet this requirement are known as USP modified lanolins.

The existing studies of hydrogel dressing versus modified lanolin (though small in number and sample sizes) show slight-to-no advantages to the hydrogel dressings in relative pain scores and healing times, showing modified lanolins to be a reasonable treatment choice for sore nipples (Brent et al., 1998; Dodd & Chalmers, 2003).

Lansinoh HPA®

Figure 9. Lansinoh®

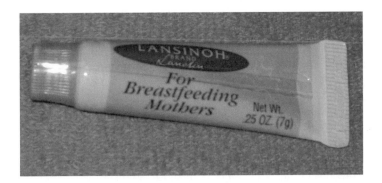

Lansinoh® HPA (for HyPoAllergenic) (figure 9) Lanolin for Breastfeeding Mothers is an ultra purified lanolin, exceeding USP specifications for modified lanolin. Lansinoh HPA's manufacturer, Lansinoh Labs, guarantees that pesticides, detergent residues, and free wool alcohols are removed, and even persons allergic to wool can use this product. The purification process involves repeated filtration and removal of volatile organic compounds so that the resulting product is odorless and tasteless. Lansinoh HPA is thick and viscous, but still allows controlled transmission of air and moisture in and out of the wound, promoting moist wound healing. The thick, viscous nature is important for the pain relieving qualities of lanolin, coating exposed free nerve endings.

Use

Mothers should wash their hands before handling their breasts or touching broken skin. A pea sized amount of Lansinoh is squeezed out of the tube onto a fingertip and gently touched to the nipple wound until it adheres. The wound and a small surrounding area should be completely covered with Lansinoh as often as needed to prevent desiccation and scab formation. The nipple can then be covered with a nursing pad (soft, finely woven cotton, wool, or smooth disposable pads are helpful to increase comfort) or breast shell to keep the Lansinoh off the clothing and further protect the nipple. Lansinoh HPA does not need to be removed before the next feeding, but use on a large area of the areola may make the breast slippery and impede latch if the baby feeds soon after application, before it is sufficiently absorbed.

Price

$10 per 2 oz tube ($145 wholesale for 50 - .25 oz tubes)

Contact Information

Lansinoh Laboratories http://www.lansinoh.com

1.800. 292.4794

Advantages

- Promotes moist wound healing if used consistently after feedings
- Contains no chemical preservatives or detergent residues
- Readily available in stores
- Small size (.25 oz) tubes are available, increasing affordability and reducing over-use

Disadvantages

- Rubs off on clothing. This can be overcome by using nursing pads or breast shells to keep nipples from rubbing on clothing, and by patting a small amount onto the wounded area and a millimeter or two around the wound only. Pre-treat stains with detergent before laundering.

Suggested Use

- Lansinoh HPA is good for partial and full thickness nipple wounds, and can be recommended to mothers with vasospasm.

Medela Purelan 100

Purelan 100 is purified by heat treatment, which removes all but traces of the free lanolin alcohols and pesticides. It has a slight odor and a deeper color than Lansinoh HPA. It is similarly well tolerated by mothers with wool allergy

Use

A pea sized amount should be squeezed onto a very clean finger and patted onto the sore nipple and a small (1-2mm) margin surrounding the wound after breastfeeding. Covering the PureLan with a soft nursing pad or breast shell will reduce the risk of staining the bra.

Price

$10 per 2 oz tube

Contact Information

Medela, Inc. http://www.medelabreastfeedingus.com/

1.800.435.8316

Advantages

- Promotes moist wound healing if used consistently after feeding

Disadvantages

- May stain clothing (reduce risk by covering treated nipples with smooth nursing pad or shells and pre-treat stains with detergent before laundering.)
- Is not in Medela's 2009 catalog

Suggested Uses

- Use for partial to full thickness nipple wounds
- May be used by mothers with vasospasm

Medela Tender Care Lanolin

Figure 10. Medela Tender Care™ Lanolin

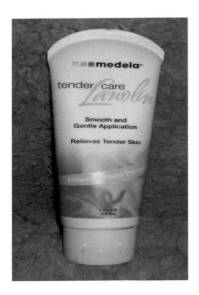

Tender Care™ Lanolin (figure 10) is heat purified like Purelan, and then has medium chain triglycerides (MCT oil) added to increase spreadability and ability to remove product from the tube in colder environments. Beta glucan micronized powder is added, as research on non-nipple skin shows this compound can enhance healing (LeBlanc et al., 2006; Wei et al., 2002; Delatte et al., 2001) by increasing activity of immune cells and increasing collagen formation and deposition (Wei et al., 2002). No research has been done on the effect of incidental ingestion of beta glucan by a breastfed infant, and Tender Care Lanolin has not been tested on injured nipples to see if it does enhance healing.

MCT's are on the FDA's list of "Generally Recognized as Safe" substances, but are not normally found in high levels in human milk, which has larger numbers of long chain fatty acids. However, babies with chylothorax (an injury to the thoracic duct that causes lymph-carrying longer chain fatty acids to build up around the heart) have been successfully fed skimmed human milk with MCT oil added as their sole fat source. One elemental manufactured milk (Pregestimil) contains MCTs as the major source of lipids.

No information is available on incidental consumption of beta glucans by infants. However, grain cell walls (particularly oats), black algae, and fungi (yeast and mushrooms) are rich in beta glucans. Human macrophages and fibroblasts contain receptors for specific beta glucans (Kougias et al., 2001; Lavigne et al., 2006), and human umbilical cord blood contains placentally-transferred IgG antibodies to several specific beta glucans (Ikewaki et al., 2007). This data taken together indicates that beta glucans are innate immune system infection recognition molecules. Indeed, beta glucans are potent immunomodulators (Gerosa et al., 2008; Luhm et al., 2006; Tsikitis et al., 2004; LeBlanc et al., 2006). More research needs to be done to fully characterize the complex interactions of beta glucan with the human immune system. However, beta glucan has been used in topical skin treatments for adults without reported adverse effects.

Use

Can be used exactly like other modified lanolins. Consider applying sparingly and gently wiping excess off before breastfeeding.

Price

$10 per 2 oz tube, $4 per .3 oz tube ($5 and $2 wholesale, respectively)

Contact Information

Medela, Inc. http://www.medelabreastfeedingus.com/

1.800.435.8316

Advantages

- Easy to spread
- Contains lower levels of pesticides and free lanolin alcohols due to dilution of USP modified lanolin (PureLan) with other ingredients

Disadvantages

- Untested on nipple skin (though FDA considers ingredients generally recognized as safe)

Suggested Use

- For mothers who find patting on thicker modified lanolins difficult or painful, consider wiping off before breastfeeding.

Alternatives to Nipple Dressings

Simply having skilled assistance with positioning and latch reduced maternal pain as rapidly as skilled assistance combined with modified lanolin (Lansinoh) used with breast shells (Ameda) or with glycerin gel dressings (Soothies) (Cadwell et al., 2004). However, there was a trend toward maternal preference for the glycerin gel pads. This still leaves a reasonable proportion of mothers who preferred Lansinoh and breast shells. The age-old practice of expressing milk onto sore nipples and allowing it to dry can be used as well. Hand hygiene (washing with soap and water) is vital before touching injured nipples to avoid introducing pathogens to broken skin.

Honey Dressings

Honey has traditionally been used on wounds by many cultures for its antibacterial properties and moist wound healing activity. Honey stimulates macrophages to release important growth factors (Tonks et al., 2001) and cytokines, particularly IL-1-beta and IL-6 (Tonks et al., 2003). IL-6 stimulates reproduction of keratinocytes and is vital for the final stages of healing. Honey, like human milk, contains sugars that prevent bacterial adhesion to tissues, preventing colonization and biofilm production (Lerrer et al., 2007). Manuka honey dressing is recommended for reducing bacterial loads in infected wounds in a British dermatology textbook (Ashton & Leppard, 2004, p 35). German midwives commonly use honey to treat infected nipples, according to Elien Rouw, MD (personal communication, December 18, 2008).

Topical application of honey has produced wound closure in case reports and series of infected wounds that resisted healing for several months to three years, including those infected with MRSA (Cooper et al., 2001; Visavadia et al., 2008; Simon et al., 2006). Though raw honey can contain Clostridium botulinum spores which can theoretically cause infant botulism if ingested (Tanzi & Gabay, 2002; Cox & Hinkle, 2002), no adverse consequences of topical honey were reported in a large case series of 59 (Efem, 1988). Indeed, untreated topical honey has been used safely and successfully in a series of 9 neonates with non-healing infected surgical wounds, eliminating the infection within 7 days (Vardi et al., 1998), even in the 6 infants whose systemic antibiotics were discontinued at the start of honey therapy.

Heat sterilization of honey destroys the antimicrobial activity as well as the complex carbohydrate responsible for stimulating cytokines (Tonks et al., 2007). To remove any potential for bacterial spore survival, medical honey is gamma irradiated to destroy spores without affecting medically useful biological activity (Molan & Allen, 1996).

Contraindications

Honey dressings should not be used if honey or bee product (or bee sting) allergy exists.

Medihoney™

Figure 11. Medihoney™ 100% medical grade sterilized honey

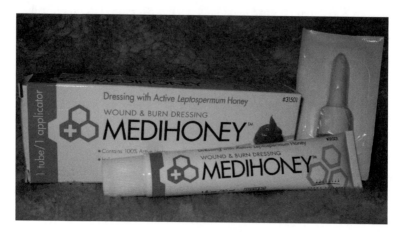

Medihoney™ is Manuka honey from New Zealand that is collected and processed under standardized conditions. It is sterilized by gamma irradiation to kill any bacterial spores and is packed sterile in 30g tubes of 100% honey, and 25g tubes of 80% honey gel (with natural waxes and oils as the other ingredients). The 100% honey version is completely water soluble and is most suitable for use on nipple wounds, as any residue can be gently rinsed off before breastfeeding. Medihoney is FDA approved as a wound dressing and unlike occlusive hydrogel dressings is suitable for use on infected or chronic (non-healing) wounds. While not yet FDA approved as an antimicrobial, evidence is mounting that Medihoney is active against a variety of pathogens. Other developed countries have certified it for use as a topical antimicrobial.

While many different honeys tested were active against most bacteria, Manuka honey was more active than most. It was particularly effective against Staph aureus (Lusby et al., 2005), an organism that is a frequent cause of nipple and breast infection, Manuka honey is more effective than other tested honeys in quenching tissue-damaging oxygen free-radicals (Henriques et al., 2006), which may be another mechanism that enhances healing. In an RCT of Medihoney versus mupirucin at catheter port sites in 101 hemodialysis patients, there were similar numbers of infections in both groups, but no facilitation of microbial resistance in the Medihoney group (Johnson et al., 2005). With the greater incidence of methicillin resistant Staph aureus (MRSA) mastitis in lactating women and the knowledge that organisms enter the breast through injured nipples, a treatment that bacteria do not seem to develop resistance to is potentially very useful.

While Medihoney is indicated for chronic as well as acute wounds, chronic nipple wounds should be followed closely by a physician to rule out Paget's disease of the breast, an uncommon form of breast cancer. (The entire phrase Paget's disease of the breast is important to avoid confusion with Paget's disease of bone, an unrelated condition). Paget's disease of the breast initially looks like a sore nipple, but it does not heal with treatment and will persist after weaning. The longer the cancer is allowed to persist in the nipple, the greater the chance that solid tumors will develop in the breast. The prognosis for any cancer is better the earlier it is identified.

Figure 12. Paget's disease of the breast

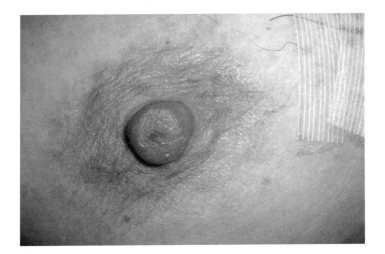

Use

After breastfeeding, wash hands carefully and apply a 3 mm deep film of Medihoney to the wound and a 1-2 mm margin around it. Cover with a nursing pad or similar absorbent dressing. Rinse with warm water before breastfeeding to remove any residue. Reapply after each breastfeeding. Expect substantial to total healing within 5 days.

Price

$9 per one ounce tube wholesale, $15-30 retail

Contact Information

Derma Sciences http://www.dermasciences.com

1.800.445.7627

Advantages

- Natural product, may appeal more to breastfeeding mothers than technological dressings

- Sterile

- Multiple mechanisms of action (moist wound healing, low (3.5) pH, high osmolality, specific antimicrobials, stimulates macrophages to release cytokines and growth factors, strong autolytic debridement, enzymatic debridement, releases hydrogen peroxide, quenches free radicals).

- Antimicrobial

Disadvantages

- No specific research has been done on lactating nipples, but is generally recognized as safe and approved for over the counter sale by the FDA

- Requires a secondary dressing (nursing pad or gauze)

- Sticky to apply, may be difficult to rinse off (hold clean washcloth dampened with warm water to nipple until honey melts and sloughs off)

Suggested Uses

- Partial to full thickness wounds, infected wounds, and wounds at risk of infection.

- May be the best amorphous dressing for very painful wounds, as its viscous nature protects the wound from air and friction.

Figure 13. Late stage Paget's disease. This nipple lesion was associated with a 10 cm tumor in the breast.

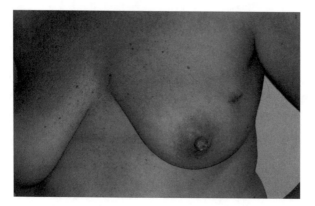

Film dressings – 3M™ Tegaderm ™

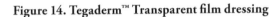

Figure 14. Tegaderm™ Transparent film dressing

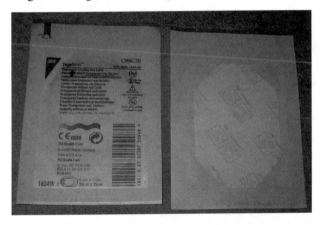

Transparent film dressing can be used to protect newly healed skin which has only 20% of the tensile strength of intact skin (Okan et al., 2007). Lactating breasts usually leak milk through surgical wounds, which can help prevent infection, but might slightly retard the speed of healing. This is not a problem if the wound is far enough from the nipple that the baby's mouth does not cover it. For wounds that are nearer the nipple, use of a transparent film dressing over the incision site might allow the mother to breastfeed directly or improve her comfort during pumping.

Transparent film dressings can be used to cover incision and drainage sites to prevent wound fluids from entering milk during pumping. Rene Fisher, BA, IBCLC, and I worked with a breastfeeding mother after incision and drainage of a periareolar abscess. Pumping was painful and resulted in purulent material leaking from the wound into the milk. The mother and infant's healthcare providers strongly cautioned against giving the infant this milk. Since the contralateral breast was producing insufficient milk to provide all of the infant's calories, the mother needed to use milk from the affected breast as well. Tegaderm™ transparent film dressing was used to cover the incision site and both improved the comfort of pumping by splinting the incision and prevented wound drainage from entering the milk (Figure 15). Note that the pump flange fit is tight, larger flanges were supplied for the next expression, which improved comfort and milk yield further.

Figure 15. Using Tegaderm™ over a small dressing to improve pumping safety and comfort after abscess drainage surgery

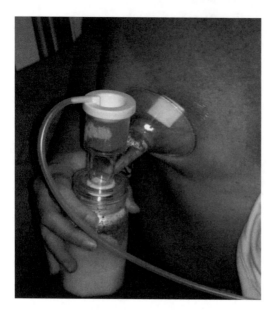

Use

Apply directly over a newly healed wound, or over a primary dressing (gauze pad) for open wounds.

Price

Less than $1 each, about 37 cents wholesale.

Contact Information

3M 1.888.3M HELPS

http://solutions.3m.com/wps/portal/3M/en_US/SH/SkinHealth/brands/tegaderm/

Advantages

- Available in single quantities
- Individually sterile packed
- Semi-permiable (allows some air through but blocks liquids)

Disadvantages

- Not for use on nipples

Suggested Uses

- For protection of newly healed non-nipple breast wounds or covering surgical wounds in the lactating breast to prevent wound fluids from entering the infant's mouth or expressed milk.

- May also make breastfeeding or pumping more comfortable by splinting the wound.

Figure 16 illustrates characteristics of the various products discussed in table format for easier comparison.

Figure 16. Relevant characteristics of the various nipple healing products

Category	Product	Water vapor transmission	Absorption	Indications	Special features	Use	Cautions
Hydrogels-amorphous	Derma Sciences AquaSite	High	Low	Deep or shallow wounds	Contours well to wound	Apply 1-2 mm beyond wound edges, cover, rinse off before feeding	May not be suitable for infected wounds
Hydrogel with Alginate, amorphous	ConvaTec Saf-Gel	High	Moderate	Deep or shallow wounds	Higher absorption for leaking breasts or wounds	Apply 1-2 mm beyond wound edges, cover, rinse off before feeding	May not be suitable for infected wounds
Hydrogel Pad	Ameda Comfort Gel Pads	High	Low	Shallow to full thickness wounds	Greater friction protection Clinically tested on lactating nipples	Rinse, apply, remove and rinse breast before feeding	Not for use on infected wounds
Hydrogel Pad	Maternal Concept Cooling Care Hydrogel Pads	High	Low	Shallow wounds, burns	Greater cooling	Apply, remove pad for feeding	Short duration of use, several hours
Hydrogel Pad	Medela Tender Care Hydrogels	High	Low	Shallow wounds	Tackier than most	Rinse, shake, let sit 2 minutes, rinse breast before feeding	Not for use on infected wounds

Hydrogel Pad	Soothies	High	Low	Shallow wounds	Contains glycerin, controls bacteria in the pad Clinically tested on lactating nipples	Apply, remove and rinse breast before feeding	Not for use on infected wounds
USP Lanolin	Lansinoh HPA	High	Low	Shallow to full thickness wounds	No need to rinse before feeding Clinically tested on lactating nipples	Wash hands, soften between fingers, dab on	May be used over antifungal ointment
USP Lanolin	Medela Purelan	High	Low	Shallow to full thickness wounds	No need to rinse before feeding	Wash hands, soften between fingers, dab on	Infected wounds?
USP Lanolin with additives	Medela Tender Care Lanolin	?	Low		Contains medium chain triglyceride oil and beta glucans	Apply sparingly, consider washing off before feeding	Infected wounds?
Medical Grade Honey	MediHoney	High	High	Shallow to full thickness wounds, infected wounds	Antibacterial activity comparable to mupirocin ointment, gamma irradiated to kill spores	Wash hands, apply sparingly, rinse with water before feeding	Chance of stinging sensation (15%)
Film Dressings	Tegaderm	Moderate	None	Breast wounds (incision and drainage, biopsy sites)	Supports newly healed skin's low tensile strength, prevents milk leakage	Wash and dry area, apply, leave on 24 hours or more	Not for use on nipples

Nipple Everters

Inverted nipples are a risk factor for suboptimal breastfeeding (Dewey et al., 2003). Even in Indonesia, a culture with 97% breastfeeding initiation, inverted nipples are cited as a barrier to breastfeeding (Suharyono & Paul, 1997). When the nipple fails to separate from the underlying gland during development, the ducts through the nipple do not lengthen normally, and even surgical treatment frequently fails to correct them (Terrill & Stapleton, 1991). Unfortunately, tools and techniques that were commonly used to bring out inverted nipples (Hoffman exercises and breast shells) have been shown in a large multicenter randomized clinical trial not to improve breastfeeding rates (Alexander et al., 1992). Breast shells used prenatally were responsible for breast and nipple infections and other adverse outcomes, and were associated with decreased breastfeeding success (MAIN Trial Collaborative Group, 1994).

Nipple problems that have different causes require different solutions. Tethered nipples are inverted nipples that cannot evert with stimulation, temporary traction, or suction. Flat nipples can either be due to less muscle tone in the muscles that evert the nipple, in which case stimulation will evert them, or to shortened ducts that tether them. Pseudoinverted nipples appear inverted, but evert with stimulation, and other than a propensity for fungal infection if allowed to invert while still damp, function well. If a nipple does not evert with a pump, into a nipple shield, or after reverse pressure softening, it is likely tethered. If nipples are flat or pseudoinverted due to muscular imbalance, temporary suction devices are likely to help. If nipples are tethered, sustained suction over a substantial period of time (weeks to months) will be required for correction.

Tools that have been shown to be effective in increasing nipple eversion in small studies and case series rely on suction. Several different modified syringe tools have been devised. The simplest is a 10 or 20 ml syringe with the tip end cut off and the plunger replaced through the cut end (Arsenault, 1997). In a small study of this tool, 7 of 8 mothers of failure to thrive infants were able to breastfeed and restore milk production within 4-6 weeks of beginning its use (Arsenault, 1997; Kesaree et al., 1993). A twin syringe device, using a 5 ml syringe and a 10 ml syringe attached by the luer slip tips with a short length of snugly fitted tubing, requires no cutting (Ozcan & Kahveci, 1995). A commercial version of the inverted syringe tool is sold by Maternal Concepts as the Evert-it.

Inverted syringes are less effective for tethered nipples (inverted nipples with shortened ducts) because pressure cannot be maintained for long enough to provide a growth stimulus to lengthen them. The Nipplette™ was designed to overcome this problem (McGeorge, 1994), but cannot be used during the third trimester of pregnancy or postpartum as the negative pressure causes milk release, filling the empty space in the device cup and eliminating the vacuum. If a woman has difficulty breastfeeding due to tethered nipples, she can be informed that this device can be used before or early in her next pregnancy. Childless young women sometimes also consult LCs for solutions to inverted nipples that will not impair future breastfeeding.

Supple Cups™ are a new and inexpensive alternative for producing sustained suction on tethered nipples that can be used during breastfeeding. Unlike syringe based alternatives, they are unlikely to produce excessive and uncomfortable suction. Supple Cups are a new product, and clinical research is ongoing. Julie Bouchet-Horwitz, FNP-BC, IBCLC, is preparing a case series for publication. She trialed Supple Cups in 13 pregnant and lactating women with inverted and flat nipples. Julie found that Supple Cups are effective for inverted nipples if worn from 37 weeks of pregnancy until delivery, as tolerated. Her clients started with half an hour per day and increased to about 4 hours per day of use, and all were able to breastfeed postpartum. Mothers with flat nipples were advised to wear the Supple Cups for several minutes before each breastfeeding and found that the cups improved infant latch.

Other devices that work on temporary vacuum have been developed for treatment of flat or inverted nipples. The Evert-It™ Nipple Enhancer by Maternal Concepts® consists of a modified (open front) syringe that fits into a reversible silicone nipple cup. One side of the cup is for smaller diameter nipples, the reverse side is for larger diameter nipples. The manufacturer did an internet based survey of their users and found that even without use between feedings as recommended, 95% of respondents found the device effective after 1-5 uses.

Lansinoh® markets a tiny bulb syringe device called the LatchAssist™ that is designed for use for flat nipples due to engorgement. It is used right before feeding to draw out the nipple. The LatchAssist is based on the same principle as using a breast pump briefly, but it is more convenient. The opening measures less than 2 cm, so it is appropriate for fairly small nipples. This is a new product, and no studies have been performed yet. The few women who have used it in my own practice have found it to be comfortable and easy to use with one hand, but the nipple only remains everted very briefly.

Alternatives

Some women can work out their inverted nipples with their fingertips, and then attach the infant. Infants can learn to breastfeed without an everted nipple, particularly if they have good tongue mobility to grasp the breast (the tongue comes down and forward to grasp the breast when the baby opens wide to latch). A short period (several feedings to several days) of cup or spoon feeding can teach the baby that feeding can occur without something firm in the mouth (page 161). Brief use of a breast pump may improve nipple protractility temporarily so the baby can attach more easily. A supplementer may both give the baby a latch cue (see supplementers) and an instant reward for attempting to attach. Babies with limited tongue mobility should be assessed for tongue-tie or neurologically based sucking difficulties, and those issues addressed.

Specific Devices to Evert Nipples

Inverted Syringe

An inexpensive nipple everter can be made from an inverted syringe. Match the diameter of the mother's nipple with the open end of the syringe, where the plunger inserts. Remove the plunger and cut off the end of the syringe that connects to the needle. Reassemble the syringe with the plunger in the cut end.

Use

The uncut end of the syringe is placed against the nipple and moistened with clean water or milk to improve adherence to the breast. The plunger is pulled out gently, enough so that the nipple is pulled forward, but not so much that there is pain. If milk is released, it will fill some of the space in the syringe and reduce the suction. If this occurs, the plunger can be pulled out a little more. The syringe is removed by breaking the seal by pressing a finger at the base of the nipple. The infant is immediately offered the breast.

Price

Less than $1, depending on size of syringe.

Contact Information

Many medical and veterinary supply companies sell syringes without needles. In some states, only physicians may purchase syringes from medical supply firms. http://www.grogans.com/ carries a wide range of syringes.

Advantages

- Inexpensive
- Readily available in health care settings
- Different capacity syringes can be modified to provide a more individualized fit

Disadvantages

- Modifying tools or using them for other than their intended use may expose one to legal liability
- Remarkably difficult to cut syringes with hand tools
- May theoretically increase the risk of preterm labor in pregnant women before 37 weeks gestation

Suggested Uses

- Useful immediately before feeding to help draw out the nipple for an infant who will not attach otherwise.

Dual Syringe

Figure 17. Dual syringe, syringes connected by aquarium tubing

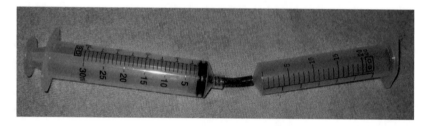

A 5ml luer slip syringe is attached to a 10 ml luer slip syringe by a short length of tubing or coupler such that the tips of the syringes are attached to each other. Aquarium tubing or IV tubing may be used as a coupler as long as it fits snugly over the syringe ends. Commercially produced "female" luer couplers are also available, in lug, thread, and elbow styles to hold the two syringes together at the tips without allowing air to escape.

Use

The plunger is removed from the smaller syringe, and the syringe opening is placed against the nipple area. The plunger is then withdrawn on the larger syringe until the nipple everts. The suction is broken with a finger at the nipple, and the infant is immediately offered the breast.

Price

About $1, including both syringes and tubing

Contact Information

Couplers are available from http://www.valueplastics.com/products/luer_fittings.aspx or http://westernfluids.net (Connex item # CX-021 and CX-027) Syringes are available from any medical supplier, including http://www.grogans.com/

Advantages

- Requires less modification than the inverted syringe
- Inexpensive

Disadvantages

- More difficult to use alone, the outer syringe is difficult to stabilize so the plunger can be withdrawn

Suggested Uses

- Temporary use in environments such as hospitals that do not allow modification of tools. Since all components of this tool are commercially available as is, and similar couplers are frequently used on IV tubing, it may be more defensible.

Evert-it™ Nipple Enhancer

Figure 18. Evert-it™ Nipple Enhancer

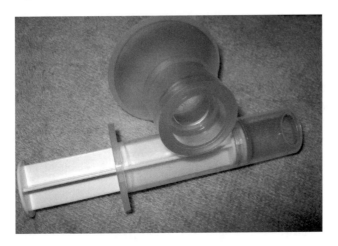

Available from Maternal Concepts, this modified inverted syringe has a soft cup (cone) at the nipple end, which is reversible to provide two different sizes. The cone has a partition molded into the interior of the smaller end. A syringe barrel fits into the cone and can either stop at the partition or be pushed beyond it to provide more pressure. The syringe plunger has a detachable non-latex seal which does not decompose when washed with dish detergents (unlike syringes manufactured for injection or irrigation use). The manufacturer cites that survey respondents found the device very effective (69%) or somewhat effective (21%), but fails to reveal the number of users surveyed, the number of non-responders, or the design of the survey.

Use

Detach the soft silicone cone from the syringe and choose the side which fits comfortably over the nipple. Attach the syringe barrel into the cone, pressing until it is firmly seated (when used with the larger side against the breast, pressure can be increased by pressing the syringe barrel farther into the cone, and decreased by keeping it behind the partition). When the cone is used with the smaller side against the breast, the suction will be more intense because air is being evacuated from a much smaller space. Counsel mothers to pull the plunger of the syringe back slowly and reverse if there is any discomfort. Once a comfortable and effective suction level is reached (the nipple everts), leave the device in place for several seconds. Release the suction by pushing the plunger back in and remove. Immediately latch the baby. The Evert-it can be used up to 3 times before each latch, and between feedings, as well, to improve nipple protractility. After use, all parts should be disassembled and washed with hot soapy water, rinsed, and air dried before storage in the supplied case.

Price

$16.30 + shipping

Contact Information

Maternal Concepts http://www.maternalconcepts.com/

1.800.310.5817

Advantages

- Available commercially, designed for use on inverted or flat nipples
- The soft cup may make it more comfortable to use, and makes it easier to release suction.
- Easy to clean and comes with a storage tube to help maintain sanitary conditions and prevent loss of parts.

Disadvantages

- Relatively expensive, but reusable
- Not available in most health care settings in the vital early days of breastfeeding
- Requires two hands for use (or a relatively large hand that can stabilize the cup by pressing on the syringe body and pull the plunger at the same time

Suggested Uses

- Ideal for repeated or frequent use

Niplette™

Figure 19. Niplette™, photo courtesy of Lisa Marasco

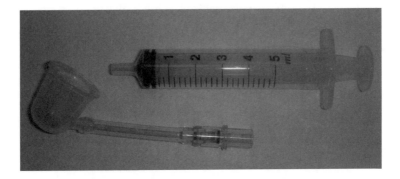

Figure 20. Niplette™ assembled, photo courtesy of Lisa Marasco

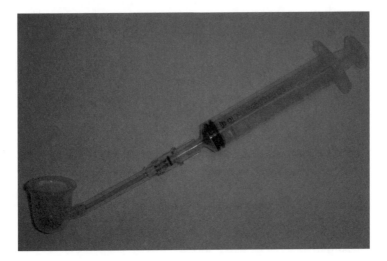

The Niplette™ (figures 19 and 20) consists of a small hard plastic cup with a short tube containing a one way valve. The cup is placed over the nipple, and a syringe is attached to the tube to evacuate air until the nipple everts. The syringe is then removed, and the cup is worn for as long as desired, optimally at least 8 hours per day. The evidence for the effectiveness of the Niplette comes from a case series published by the device's developer (McGeorge, 1994). Used between pregnancies or during early to mid pregnancy, the device provided long term negative pressure on the nipple and could be worn under loose clothing or during sleep. The sustained negative pressure is postulated to put directional stress on the tissues of the ducts to cause them to grow (lengthen), a hypothesis that is consistent with established techniques of medical tissue expansion in other human tissues. McGeorge reports that the Niplette allows permanent correction of the everted nipple. The device worked for most women in two to four months. Most impressively, all 14 women who used the device during pregnancy were able to breastfeed, including six for whom breastfeeding failed with previous infants. The Niplette is distributed by Philips Avent.

Use

Place rigid plastic cup over nipple, attach syringe to stem. Pull out plunger until nipple everts, reduce suction by pushing back plunger if discomfort results. Detach syringe, leave in place as tolerated, up to eight hours a day. Use daily during early pregnancy or between pregnancies until permanent nipple eversion occurs. Retain device for booster use if nipple retracts again. Should not be used during the last trimester of pregnancy or during lactation, as it is less effective and may theoretically increase the risk of preterm labor.

Price

The kit of two devices (one for each nipple) retails for around $50/£30

Contact Information

Philips Avent 1.203.351.5000

Advantages

- May provide permanent correction, but relapse after discontinuation and treatment failure in some cases reported on mothering forums
- Permits normal breastfeeding when it works

Disadvantages:

- Cannot be used during lactation as the device loses suction as it fills with milk
- Relatively expensive
- Uncomfortable rigid cup and tube
- Not readily available, but can be ordered online

Suggested For

- Young women who want a treatment that will preserve the ability to breastfeed
- Women who have had breastfeeding difficulties with prior children due to tethered nipples

Supple Cups™

Figure 21. Supple Cups™

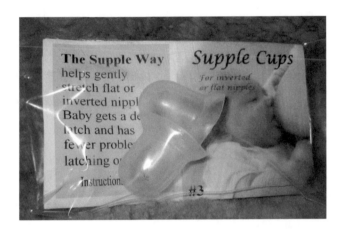

These soft silicone cups are squeezed between two fingers at the closed end, then the open rim is gently pressed against the base of the nipple, and the pressure released. The manufacturer recommends lubricating the nipple and the Supple Cup's rim with a little Lansinoh® to reduce friction on the skin and to help them adhere. Using modified lanolin is especially important if they are to be worn for more than a few minutes to prevent leaking milk from dislodging the cups. The baby can be fed dripped colostrum from the cup after removal if desired. If an inverted nipple will come out with use of the Supple Cup, but will not stay everted, Julie Bouchet-Horowitz recommends first using the Supple Cup, then immediately applying a nipple shield to maintain the nipple in an everted position.

If the mother wishes to wear a bra, she may need to wear breast shells over the Supple Cup to avoid uncomfortable pressure, as they project out over the breast surface. Wholesale pricing of $7 per pair (10 pairs minimum) is available to LCs who wish to give or resell these to their clients, or $6.50 per pair in lots of 50 pairs for hospitals. Three sizes are available, see chart.

Table 1. Breast Shell Sizes

Size	Interior Diameter	
#2	½ inch	12.7 mm
#3	9/16 inch	14.3 mm
#4	5/8 inch	15.9 mm

Use

Wash hands with soap and water. Lubricate rim of Supple Cup with a small amount of modified lanolin, squeeze top with fingers, and apply to breast, being careful to center it around the nipple, press in toward breast gently, release pressure from fingers. Wear several minutes before feeding for postpartum use. If used between pregnancies or during the last three weeks of gestation, work up to wearing several hours a day. Supple Cups may be covered with a breast shell, if desired, to prevent pressure on cup from bra. If a breast shell is used, make sure bra is loose enough to avoid putting undue pressure on the breast. Wash with hot soapy water, rinse, and air dry between uses. Figures 22-26 illustrate the use and effectiveness of Supple Cups.

Figure 22. Spreading lanolin on the rim of the supple cup

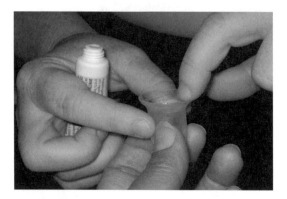

Figure 23. Flat nipple

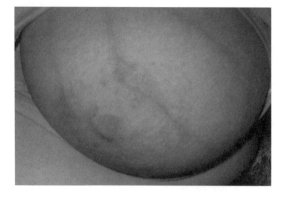

Figure 24. Applying Supple Cup

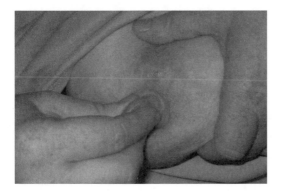

Figure 25. Supple Cup in place

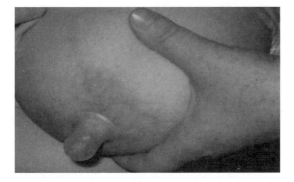

Figure 26. Nipple after 2 minutes in Supple Cup.

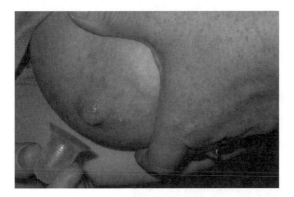

Price

$14.95/pair retail; $7/pair wholesale with minimum order of 10; $6.50/50 pair for hospitals

Contact Information

http://www.supplecups.com sales@supplecups.com

Advantages

- Inexpensive
- Soft and comfortable for most women
- Simple to apply
- Effective
- Available in multiple sizes to fit different diameter nipples

Disadvantages

- Project from the body, may be difficult to wear discreetly (can be worn at night instead)

Suggested Uses

- Works for tethered or pseudoinverted nipples
- Can be used briefly for 1-5 minutes before feeding, to evert flat or inverted nipples in early postpartum or to increase nipple eversion during engorgement
- Can be worn for increasing periods of time (30 minutes to 4 hours daily) during the last 3 weeks of pregnancy to provide sustained pressure on tethered nipples, or as long as needed between pregnancies

Lansinoh® LatchAssist™

Figure 27. LatchAssist™ in use

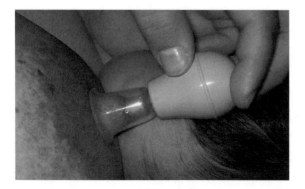

LatchAssist™ (figure 27) is a small bulb syringe attached to a plastic cup meant to surround the nipple and allow suction to be applied to temporarily evert the nipple. The use of a bulb instead of a syringe allows the device to be used with one hand. The cup is rigid plastic and relatively small, the opening is less than 20mm in diameter, so it will not fit wider nipples. It sells for about $10 at many large retailers and is available online. The device comes with a small plastic case that keeps it clean between uses, especially outside the home. In the detailed instructions, the manufacturer recommends it be used for nipples that are flattened by engorgement, but the box text reads "To help the correction of inverted or flattened nipples of the postpartum lactating mother, by everting the nipple, allowing an infant to latch-on."

Use

The instructions advise the mother to position the baby near the breast, then squeeze the bulb, press the plastic cup over the nipple to create a seal, and slowly release the bulb to provide pressure. This is to be repeated until the nipple is temporarily everted. Since the effects are temporary, a delay in latching the baby will require the process be repeated. I would recommend the LatchAssist be placed cup down after use until it can be washed to avoid milk dripping into the bulb syringe. Bulb syringe breast pumps have long been considered an infection risk due to the inability to properly clean the inside of the bulb. While it is likely that far less milk will get into the LatchAssist bulb, careful cleaning with hot soapy water and use by only one woman per device is prudent.

Price

$10

Contact Information

Lansinoh Laboratories http://www.lansinohlabs.com

1.800.292.4794

Advantages

- Can be used with one hand
- Small, simple, and portable
- Effective for nipples that are not tethered
- Inexpensive, readily available

Disadvantages

- Difficult to clean inside of bulb syringe - theoretical infection risk
- Effects are temporary and brief

Suggested Use

- Use to evert nipples immediate postpartum, especially during engorgement
- Use immediately before feedings

Alternative

- Reverse pressure softening (Cotterman, 2004)

Nipple Shields

Nipple shields have been controversial as breastfeeding tools before the very recent past. This is partially due to design issues. Early modern nipple shields consisted of a glass shield with a rubber teat attached. The teat sat way off the breast. It was useful mainly to accustom the infant to being held and sucking in a breastfeeding position, but allowed little milk transfer. More modern shields were thick rubber, with a very small opening into which the average nipple would not fit. These "Mexican hat" nipple shields reduced milk intake by 58% when used by 5-8 day old infants; the thin latex shields reduced milk intake to a lesser extent (22%) (Woolridge et al., 1980).

Current nipple shields are ultra-thin silicone. A study assessing pumping using a nipple shield found a reduction in milk volume pumped with silicone and latex shields (Auerbach, 1990). However, recent studies of breastfeeding with a thin silicone nipple shield showed normal maternal prolactin and cortisol levels and improved breastfeeding for selected infants (Chertok et al., 2006).

A chart review of 15 preterm infants unable to breastfeed for 5 days before nipple shield use (Clum & Primomo, 1996) found that all were able to transfer some milk at their first nipple shield use, and 60% were able to transfer at least half their calculated need. In this study, nipple shields were used when the infant was unable to sustain latch or had a dysfunctional suck and when the mother had flat or large nipples (Clum & Primomo, 1996). With support from IBCLCs and nurses trained to provide assistance in their absence, all but one of the 15 infants using nipple shields were breastfeeding, most exclusively and without the shield, at discharge. Informal discussion with mothers in the study revealed that they found the nipple shield reduced their frustration, and the authors speculate that this allowed continuing efforts to breastfeed. Paula Meier (Meier et al., 2000) similarly found that her study population of 34 preterm infants who had difficulty attaching or remaining attached was able to transfer more milk with a thin silicone nipple shield than without one. Longer sucking bursts and better alertness were also noted.

Barbara Wilson-Clay (Wilson-Clay, 1996) found in a chart review of 32 dyads that nipple shields were useful as a "bridge" back to breastfeeding for bottle fed infants and infants with persistent tongue tip elevation, for placing over a tube for infants requiring supplementation at breast who seemed bothered by the feel of the tube, and for mothers with flat and inverted nipples whose infants were unable to attach without the device. She cautioned that careful attention to infant growth is required when using a nipple shield. Vicky Bodley and Diane Powers instructed their clients to use an electric breast pump several times a day to protect milk production while using a nipple shield. In their follow up of 10 clients using nipple shields (Bodley & Powers, 1996), only one of the mothers pumped sporadically, the others did not pump at all, and all infants grew appropriately.

An additional use for nipple shields is to increase tactile characteristics of the breast for infants with neurological or sensory processing difficulties (Genna, 2008). Infants with these issues may root repeatedly but not attach, or might attach very briefly but be unable to maintain their latch. The nipple shield can help maintain the nipple in the mouth of an infant with low muscle tone between sucks and can make a more definite "latch here" cue for an infant with reduced sensory awareness.

A nipple shield can also be useful in transitioning the infant who shows breast distress from bottle to breast by using a "bait and switch" technique (Genna, 2008, p. 260). The mother applies a nipple shield, and the infant is bottle fed in a breastfeeding position, as close to the breast as possible. The infant is brought into alignment to latch to the breast as the bottle is removed. Most infants will latch onto the breast and suck at least a few times. If the infant is unwilling to suck until the milk ejection reflex (MER) occurs, the nipple shield can be pre-filled with expressed milk or artificial milk with a curved tip syringe (figure 28).

Maternal issues may also indicate the use of a nipple shield. Diane Powers and Vicky Bodley Tapia retrospectively surveyed 202 mothers in their practice who had used nipple shields during the previous 3 years (Powers & Tapia, 2004). They found that maternal reasons were as common as infant issues in the decision to use a shield: 69% used a shield to allow their infant to latch to their flat nipples, and 23% used the shield to relieve nipple soreness during breastfeeding. In all, 88% of the mothers felt the nipple shield contributed to their breastfeeding success. Powers and Tapia write:

> *"It is of equal importance for lactation consultants to interpret the individual mother's ability to cope with pain or frustration. Women with low pain tolerance or frustration levels may default to formula if other solutions are not provided quickly enough for them" (p. 330-331).*

Figure 28. A curved tip syringe fits into the holes of the nipple shield. Once the shield is firmly placed, it can be pre-filled with milk to encourage a reluctant nurser.

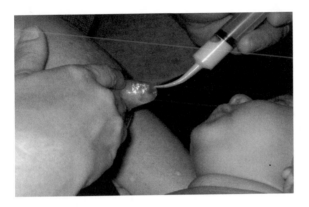

Sizing Nipple Shields

The size of nipple shield that is useful depends on how it is applied and how the infant latches to it (taking just the teat or taking some of the flat portion around the teat, and thus more breast tissue). If a larger shield is used and a significant amount of breast tissue beyond the nipple can be drawn into the teat, the infant needs to take less of the breast beyond the teat. If a small nipple shield is used, it is unlikely that much more than the maternal nipple can fit in the teat; so the infant must take more than just the teat in the mouth to feed effectively. The fit of the teat must also allow expansion of the maternal nipple, which in turn allows expansion of the nipple ducts to release milk. A very tight fit between the shield and maternal nipple is like a too small breast pump nipple tunnel, and may impede milk release the same way. If nipple blood flow is interrupted (the nipple turns purple or has a white ring at the base), the shield is probably too narrow.

The nipple generally lengthens during sucking and may contact the top of the teat. If the nipple has impressions from the holes in the tip of the teat after the baby suckles, the teat is too short for that dyad.

The nipple shield must also fit the infant mouth. If the nipple shield teat is longer than the infant palate, it will reinforce shallow attachment at the breast and will usually greatly reduce milk transfer. A shallow latch can also expose the maternal nipple to the infant's gums, which will still hurt through the nipple shield. Unfortunately, nipple shields with wider diameters at the base also have longer teats, so fitting both mother and baby optimally may be impossible. Sometimes the breastfeeding problem is the infant's inability to handle the maternal nipple diameter, which is not remediable with a shield (Wilson-Clay & Hoover, 2005, p. 58). Finding the best compromise in size for each dyad may require some experimentation. It is not unreasonable to try a different size nipple shield briefly if the originally selected one does not work well.

Application

Lactation Consultants have invented many methods to draw the breast into a nipple shield, improving the shield's adhesion to the breast and filling out the teat portion to improve its stability during latch. Linda Pohl, PE, IBCLC, an engineer and lactation consultant, applied her engineering knowledge to the use of breastfeeding tools to find ways to optimize their use (Pohl, 2003). Her method is to shorten the nipple shield teat by pressing it into the base with the thumbs while the fingers bring the flat portion of the shield toward the teat. The remaining portion of the teat is used to gather up as much nipple tissue as possible. The mother presses a finger or two from each hand into the folded area of the shield and presses back toward her chest wall, and then angles the fingers back slightly so the teat everts and pulls the nipple and some surrounding tissue in further. It is important that the mother allows the breast to fall to its' natural position before applying the nipple shield this way, as moving the breast or nipple area will cause the breast to change shape, loosening the shield. Figures 29 through 32 illustrate Linda Pohl's technique.

Figure 29. Turning back the rim of the shield to leave only a small area of teat right-side-out

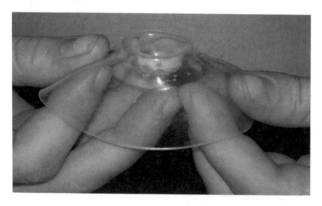

Figure 30. The shield is fitted over the nipple without lifting the breast.

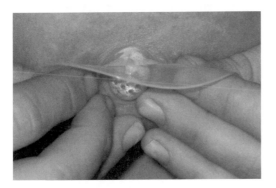

Figure 31. The fingers press the shield into the breast until the shield teat elongates, bringing the nipple and areolar tissue with it.

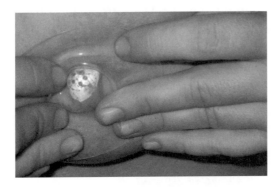

Figure 32. Ameda nipple shield in place

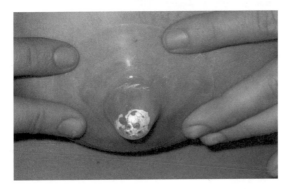

Barbara Wilson-Clay's method of applying a nipple shield is to fold the base back and stretch the base of the teat with the fingers, and then place it over the nipple and withdraw the fingers (Wilson-Clay & Hoover, 2005, p. 58). As it recoils back to its normal shape, it brings the nipple into the teat and adheres better to the breast.

Latching with the Nipple Shield

If the only way the baby can latch is to slide his lips down the nipple shield teat, this may be acceptable for the first few feedings, but once he is convinced that the breast will provide milk, he should be encouraged to latch as if the shield were not there. Positioning his chin at the base of the shield and allowing the shield teat tip to rest on his philtrum (the ridge between nose and mouth) mimics the "setup" at the bare breast for an asymmetrical latch (Genna, 2008, p. 247-8). Figure 33 illustrates this positioning at the breast with a full term baby and figure 34 shows a good latch with a nipple shield.

Figure 33. Offering the breast with a nipple shield: position baby so her chin touches the breast and the shield teat touches her philtrum, the little ridge between nose and upper lip.

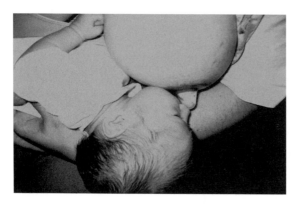

Figure 34. This baby has a significant amount of breast in her mouth below the teat of the shield, which is ideal.

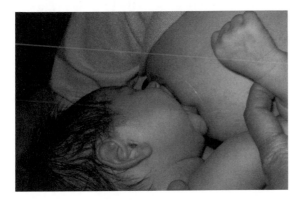

Figure 35. Alternate positioning with a nipple shield for a baby with a smaller mouth

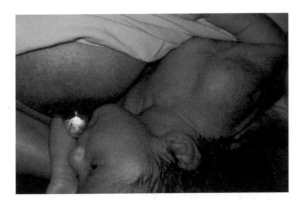

If the baby's maximal gape (mouth opening) is too small to reach over the shield teat when his chin is on the breast, both lips can be started out on the underside of the shield teat, so the sequence of the gape, bring tongue down, grasp shield, and bring upper lip over the teat that works at the bare breast is preserved. Figure 35 illustrates a good line up with a nipple shield for a smaller infant. Infants who are repeatedly allowed to slide down the teat with pursed lips are being set up for failure once the shield is removed. Sliding pursed lips along the soft human nipple pushes it out of the mouth. LCs always want to consider that any movement provides for future normal function of the infant and promote as close to normal as the infant can perform.

Evaluating Effectiveness

There are several reliable ways to assess whether an infant is transferring milk with the nipple shield in place. Test weighing before and after the feeding can be accurate if done properly on a scale designed for that use (page 109).

Assessing for suck:swallow ratio and sucking speed is also helpful. An infant transferring milk effectively will generally suck about once per second and will swallow softly once every one to two sucks. The sucks will be deep and drawing (the mandible will open, pause, close) (Newman, 2005). Faster sucking is a sign of much lower milk transfer.

When the baby releases the shield, there may be a significant pool of milk in the end of the teat or there may be milk in the infant's mouth if milk transfer was occurring (figure 36). The sated newborn will usually rest his face on the breast and close his eyes, an older baby may enter a quiet alert state and gaze up at mom. If the baby falls asleep during feeding, his behavior will indicate satiety and not just exhaustion – the fists will relax, and the baby will not immediately fuss for more food if he's laid down.

Figure 36. Baby releases breast when satiated, note milk still available in nipple shield.

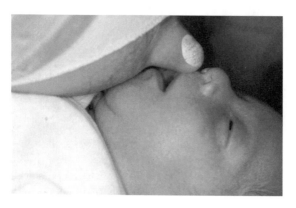

Some babies take a few practice sessions to learn to transfer milk through a nipple shield; others need a different size nipple shield to be successful. It's risky to leave a mother with a nipple shield that is not working. In carefully selected cases, the mother can be encouraged to try brief (several minutes) practice sessions at the breast with the shield as she nourishes the baby another way. A safer alternative is to work on improving the baby's feeding skills and perhaps try the nipple shield again at a follow up consultation if it is still needed. This may be particularly true of fragile babies, such as those who have been underfed or are significantly preterm or ill. Resolution of any nutritional deprivation will often lead to significant improvements in feeding behavior. Poor feeding exacerbates the nutritional deficit, and places the infant at risk. Infants who have lost more than 7-10% of birth weight or failed to gain 6-8 ounces per week during their first few months of life may benefit from supplementing at breast by a method that makes feeding less of an effort (such as with a syringe and tube) until they regain their strength.

Not all preterm infants are fragile or incapable of breastfeeding. Preterm infants differ in their capacity to produce negative intraoral pressure and are most competent if they get early access to the breast (Nyqvist, 2008). Since breastfeeding allows infants to pace the feeding, preterm infants who are capable of transferring milk from the breast generally find breastfeeding less stressful on their immature cardiorespiratory systems. For infants who cannot remove milk from the breast adequately, use of a nipple shield may increase milk transfer (Meier et al., 2000). When a nipple shield is used, milk transfer should be assessed and only infants for whom the intervention works well should continue to use it.

Maintaining Good Milk Production with a Nipple Shield

Many LCs encourage mothers using a nipple shield to pump. I originally followed the "party line" and encouraged mothers to express milk while using a nipple shield, but soon found that some mothers were developing uncomfortable hyperlactation and recurrent plugged ducts. Now instructions are individualized. If the infant feeds efficiently and effectively with the nipple shield, the mother is encouraged to watch the baby for normal energy, copious stools, and sated behaviors. If the infant is sleepier than usual, has fewer than four or five stools per day in the early weeks, or is unsettled, she is encouraged to express and feed sufficient milk to the infant to resolve these concerns. All mothers struggling with feeding problems are advised to have frequent (weekly or twice weekly) weight checks by the infant's physician. Babies with genetic, neurological, or physical conditions that may impact feeding or newborns that have lost excessive weight (over 10% of birth weight) are weighed more often.

Sometimes an experienced clinician will use a nipple shield with an infant who is not yet proficient at the breast. In this case, pumping and the provision of expressed milk in a manner that helps preserve and promote normal feeding is vital to the infant's health and the mother's continued milk production. Test weights during breastfeeding with the shield can provide information on how much the infant is getting, so that the amount of supplementation needed can be calculated. Careful follow up is needed in such cases to ensure that the infant thrives, feeding skills improve, and milk production is maintained or increased as needed.

Weaning from the Nipple Shield

Few mothers and infants continue to require a nipple shield throughout the course of breastfeeding. In my practice, only two dyads have used the shield permanently, one with bilateral inverted nipples and a tongue-tied infant, and one with maternal sensory processing difficulties.

The process of weaning off a shield depends on why the shield was used. For an infant who has had a lot of bottles and does not seem to recognize the breast as a food source, the shield might only need to be used once. When infants have a lot of frustration built up from numerous failed attempts at breastfeeding, they may require a longer period of "easy access" before being asked to work at latching again. Frequent follow up to assess the baby's attitude and behaviors can help the dyad discontinue the shield more quickly.

As soon as the infant directs normal feeding behaviors to the breast (roots, gapes, etc.), or looks excited to see the breast, weaning from the nipple shield can begin. The infant may be able to self-attach when placed for an asymmetrical latch, or the breast may need to be shaped for easier attachment. The techniques in the alternatives section (page 59) are also useful when the infant is being weaned from the nipple shield.

It may be helpful to begin weaning at a feeding when the breast is either fuller or emptier, depending on when the baby finds it easier to grasp. It may work best to offer the breast without the shield when the baby is particularly organized and calm. Some infants wean from the shield most readily if they are allowed to use the shield at the beginning of the feeding, and then it is slipped away, and they are quickly reattached to the breast. Other infants are most patient if offered the breast before they are very hungry. Babies may latch without the shield more easily if they are just awakening from a nap, particularly if mom picks them up and cuddles them to the breast before they are fully awake. In a sleepy state, the infant's reflexes may take over and allow him to have success at the breast, whereas if he were fully awake, his conditioned frustration may disorganize him so much he does not even attempt to latch. Another weaning strategy is to switch to a different nipple shield. Sometimes using a larger shield gets the infant used to taking a larger mouthful of breast. Changing nipple shields to a softer variety may be another helpful strategy. The Ameda (24 mm) shield teat is a little softer than other thin silicone nipple shields on the U.S. market, and may provide a transition between a stiffer shield and no shield at all. Medela shields become less stiff with increasing size, the 16 mm shield is very stiff, the 20 mm shield is less stiff, and the 24 mm shield is softest.

If the dyad is struggling to get rid of the shield, there are two likely issues. One is that the original reason the baby couldn't attach has not been resolved. Some infants with subtle tongue-ties will have less difficulty breastfeeding once their mouth grows a little, and they can grasp a larger mouthful of breast. Others will not improve, and the nipple shield may only mask the problem. Infants with neurological problems may gain strength and coordination with practice and may be able to move off the nipple shield, others will remain dependent on it just as they may be dependent on braces to support their leg muscles during walking. A repeat assessment and evaluation of the infant's feeding skills may highlight further interventions that may bring the infant closer to normal feeding.

The second issue that may make weaning from a nipple shield difficult is improper use. Mothers differ in their capacity to recall instructions and reproduce strategies they are taught in a consultation. Mothers may think they are offering the breast correctly, but they may be facilitating a shallow attachment to part of the teat only or may be allowing their infant to slide his lips down the shield rather than opening the mouth and grasping the breast and teat with the tongue. Taking a step backward and reinforcing good technique with the nipple shield for a few days may be all that is needed to allow transition to the bare breast.

Advantages

- Preserves at-breast feeding
- Can reduce maternal and infant frustration with breastfeeding
- Assists preterm or hypotonic infant in maintaining the nipple in the mouth, preserving energy for feeding
- Can reduce excessive negative pressure during sucking (Geddes & McClellan, 2007)

Disadvantages

- May reduce milk transfer in some infants
- Complicates feeding – can fall off repeatedly, requires cleaning, easily lost (careful application to draw up breast tissue beyond nipple into shield reduces falling off, storage in a small dedicated container reduces loss)

Alternatives to Nipple Shields

Newman (Newman, 1997) cautions that nipple shields are vulnerable to overuse and may prevent LCs from developing skills in helping babies attach and counseling mothers to be patient. Transmitting confidence that breastfeeding works and that it is a process that can take a little time for some dyads is key to helping mothers "hang on" until their infants become proficient at breastfeeding.

Exaggerated shaping of the breast with the mother's fingers or hand can often help the infant latch (Glover & Wiessinger, 2008). Some infants respond to the "breast sandwich" (Wiessinger, 1998) technique, in which the breast is flattened to match the baby's mouth, and the baby's lower lip is placed at the underside of the "sandwich." Figure 37 shows how the "breast sandwich technique" works. Note that the mother's hand is placed so it does not prevent her from holding her baby close. If shaping the breast with a hand underneath interferes with bringing the baby very close, the mother can shape her breast from the top instead, as in figures 38 and 39. This method can also help the mother not to lift her breast. When an infant has difficulty latching or staying latched, lifting the breast and then letting go may cause too much weight on the baby's jaw and tongue. Bringing the baby to where the breast naturally falls helps eliminate stress due to gravity.

Figure 37. Shaping the breast to help baby grasp a larger mouthful

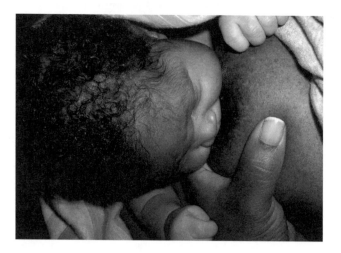

Figure 38. Shaping the breast 'from above' helps keep the hand out of the baby's way.

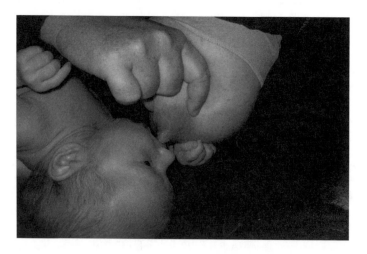

Figure 39. The mother continues to shape the breast briefly until the baby's attachment is secure.

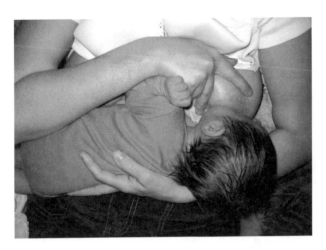

The "dent" technique (Genna, 2008) uses one fingertip pressed on the breast about an inch or two medially from the nipple to cause the areola to bulge out from the breast so the baby can dig his/her chin into the dent and grasp the bulged out areola with the tongue. The mother waits until the infant has a secure grasp on the breast before removing her finger. This technique is illustrated in figures 40 and 41. Rebecca Glover teaches moms to place a finger at the base of the nipple opposite where the baby is to latch to bulge out some of the areolar tissue to make it more graspable. The finger can be used to press additional breast into the baby's mouth as the baby begins to attach; it is slipped away as the baby attaches, flipping out the upper lip slightly if necessary (Glover, 2005). Figure 42 shows how pressing on the breast near the outer base of the nipple bulges out some breast tissue on the inner side of the nipple for the baby to grasp.

Figure 40. Denting the breast with a finger to define a mouthful can help the baby transition from a nipple shield.

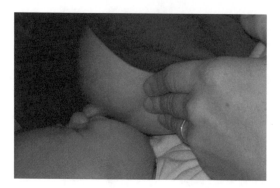

Figure 41. The mother keeps her finger on the breast until the baby has a firm grasp.

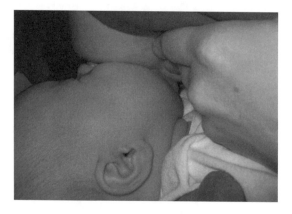

Figure 42. Defining a mouthful by pressing on the lateral aspect of the areola

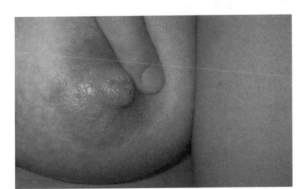

Suggested Uses for Nipple Shields:

- Use for preterm or hypotonic neurologically impaired infants who do not transfer milk well without a nipple shield.

- Use for infants who are transitioning from bottle to breast

- Use for maternal flat or inverted nipples (see nipple everters and breast shaping as alternatives)

- Use to slow milk flow to infant (check to make sure MER is excessively fast, some infants have difficulty with a normal flow, consider carefully reducing milk production if appropriate)

- Use to protect damaged nipples while mother continues to work on positioning, latch, and infant sucking problems.

Specific Products

Ameda Nipple Shield

Features

This shield is more conical than Medela's 24 mm shields, and the teat portion is the softest of the nipple shields on the market. It can be useful to gather up a large, soft nipple and in helping an infant wean off a stiffer shield. The Ameda nipple shield is pictured in figure 32.

Price

Approximately $4 wholesale, $8 retail

Contact Information

Ameda Breastfeeding Products http://www.ameda.co

1.866.99.AMEDA

Medela Nipple Shields

Features:

Medela nipple shields are available in three teat widths: 16mm, 20mm, 24mm, and in traditional and Contact™ (cut out) styles. The Contact™ shields allow the baby's chin or nose to touch the breast, depending on the orientation of the curve cut out of the shield rim. Having a variety of shield shapes and sizes can allow better adherence to the breast and better fit for the nipple or infant mouth. The more spherical the breast, the better the traditional shield shape seems to fit. The contact shield sometimes stays "put" better on a more tapered breast shape. In some dyads, the plastic rim of the nipple shield flips forward, partially blocking the infant's nose. For those dyads, the contact shield prevents this if the cutout is placed opposite the infant's nose. The teat of the 16mm shield is the firmest and is slightly shorter than the larger sizes. The 24 mm Medela Contact nipple shield is shown in use in figure 28.

Price

Approximately $4 wholesale, $8 retail

Contact Information

Medela Inc. http://www.medelabreastfeedingus.com/
1.800.435.8316

Supplementers

When maternal milk production is low or baby is unable to produce sufficient intraoral negative pressure to transfer milk well, providing additional milk to the infant during breastfeeding preserves the structural, sensory, and psychological effects of breastfeeding. The improved sucking activity at breast increases the stimulation to the breast. When milk production is low, so is flow from the breast. Many infants will not work very hard for a slow flow. The additional flow from the supplementer tube encourages more sustained sucking (longer sucking bursts and more jaw deflection), which can increase breast emptying.

This effect can be documented using a scale designed for weighing milk intake. The baby and the filled supplementer device are weighed separately. After feeding, the baby and the device are both re-weighed. The difference between the amount missing from the supplementer and the amount the baby gained is the amount the baby took directly from the breast. If the supplementer improved the baby's milk intake, increased the amount of milk he took from the breast, and did not cause respiratory or swallowing stress, it is probably a good intervention.

If the baby has difficulty coordinating swallowing and breathing with the additional milk flow, then a supplementer should not be used or one with a slower flow should be substituted. It is important to correctly assess the infant before deciding on an intervention. Babies who breastfeed with short sucking bursts (3-5 sucks per burst) are likely to have a cardiac or respiratory problem and are not usually candidates for supplementers unless their mother has a very low milk production and the supplementer will bring her up to a normal flow.

If the baby is unable to move milk from the supplementer device efficiently or if the baby takes milk ONLY from the supplementer and leaves the breast full, careful consideration should be given to discontinuing the device. Some infants take a few feedings to figure out how to get milk from the supplementer. In this case, the mother could be counseled to try using the supplementer on alternate feedings and to feed in a way that is easier for baby in between.

Babies who cannot make negative pressure in their mouths due to cleft palate or soft palate dysfunction may use a supplementer to allow feeding at the breast, even if the infant removes very little milk from the breast itself. Once the cleft is repaired, the soft palate grows, or strength and coordination improve, the baby should be able to transition to taking milk from the breast directly. Different supplementer devices require differing amounts of negative pressure to move milk from them, and some experimentation may be required to find one an infant with inadequate negative intraoral pressures can use. When used for an infant with a cleft palate, the supplementer tube may be best placed between the tongue and breast to avoid milk being delivered into the cleft and to allow for the possibility that the breast may occlude the cleft.

Using Multiple Supplementers to Increase Baby's Ability to Create Negative Intraoral Pressure

When an infant exerts insufficient negative pressure, little milk will flow from even a full breast. If milk is not removed regularly, milk production will plummet. Some LCs recommend brief breastfeeding for practice, perhaps with breast compression which increases the positive pressure in the breast and may help increase the pressure differential between the breast and the infant's mouth, without the baby needing to produce a more negative intraoral pressure (vacuum).

Supplementer devices can also be used to help an infant practice and develop negative pressure sucking. Using the therapeutic paradigm of the "just right challenge," a device that requires an amount of negative pressure that the infant can exert only with some effort is chosen. It is important to ensure that the work of feeding is not too difficult, such that the infant fails to grow appropriately (protect infant nutrition and growth). Once the infant can remove milk from the first supplementer device without much difficulty, one that requires more negative pressure can be used to increase the infant's negative pressure sucking. Infants in my practice who sucked ineffectively but were anatomically normal have benefited from this approach, and many have gone on to breastfeed exclusively and directly after two or three supplementer devices were used serially. For an infant who is a poor feeder, starting with a syringe and tube to assist the infant's efforts, and then moving to the tube in a bottle, starting with the bottle high and then moving it lower, gradually increased the infant's negative pressure sucking without requiring the mother to buy more than one device. Other mothers began with a syringe and tube and went to either an SNS™ or Lact-Aid® to challenge their infant to use negative pressure.

Choosing Between Supplementer Devices

Many different tubes can be used to provide additional milk at breast, including a 5 or 8 French feeding tube in a bottle or on a syringe, a soft dispensing tip on a syringe, "butterfly" tubing on a syringe with the needle cut off, and commercial devices - Lact-Aid® Nursing Trainer and Supplemental Nursing System™/Supply Line (Medela).

The different devices have different characteristics which make them useful in varied situations. The stiffer tubing and smooth end of a 5 French feeding tube make it ideal if the tube needs to be slipped into the corner of the infant's mouth during feeding. The stiffer tube if held or taped to the areola can also provide a "latch here" cue for the baby whose mother has flat or inverted nipples (Wiessinger, 2000). The stronger sensory quality of these stiff tubes may prove a disadvantage for a more sensitive infant. They are less desirable for use under a nipple shield, where the stiff tube can disrupt the shield's hold on the breast. The softer tube of a Lact-Aid® or SNS™ works better under a nipple shield. The tube can be placed between the nipple and partially inverted shield teat using Linda Pohl's application method (pages 52-23), and when the teat everts, it secures the tube against the breast. Figure 43 shows an infant feeding with a Lact-Aid® tube under a nipple shield.

Figure 43. Using a supplementer under a nipple shield can help infants with feeding problems be successful at the breast.

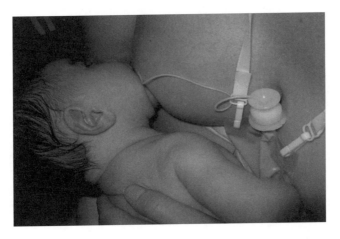

Ease of use is a consideration. A syringe and tube is inexpensive, simple to assemble, and easy to clean, but requires hand strength to provide boluses to the baby during feeding. A tube in a bottle requires no hand strength, but requires quite a bit of sucking before milk is delivered through the tube, and a reluctant baby might give up before getting a reward. A curved tip syringe is inexpensive and offers fine control of milk delivery, but can be perceived as sharp and holds only 12cc of milk. These are ideal for use as a treatment probe (to find out if giving baby extra milk at the breast will be helpful), but can be less convenient for frequent use by the mother at home. The Lact-Aid is discreet and convenient, with only the tubing to clean and a fresh, sterile bag used for each feeding. However, any time supplies are consumable, they provide a potential stressor – mom needs to reorder them to avoid running out. The SNS requires careful assembly to avoid leaking and is expensive and bulky, but it lasts a long time with careful cleaning.

When mothers are inexperienced at breastfeeding, it can be helpful for them to tape the tubing to the breast. Sterile paper first aid tape is a good choice, but falls off as soon as it gets wet. It can be challenging to tape the tubing close enough to the nipple so that the tube stays in place, yet far enough away that the tape stays dry. Most LCs teach mothers to tape along the length of the tube rather than across it, and find that wide (3/4 inch) tape works better than narrow tape. If the supplementer is going to be used at every feeding, the mother can modify a self-adhesive bandage (plaster) to hold the tubing. Use a smaller size bandage, a latex free brand with hypoallergenic glue is ideal. Cut the adhesive away from the sides of the pad, and place the bandage on the breast with the pad where the tube will go. Mother can then pinch the pad between two fingers and slide the supplementer tube underneath. The bandage can stay on the breast until the mother showers, at which time it should be removed as the pad will become wet and macerate the skin underneath. Figure 44 illustrates the use of an adhesive bandage to hold a 5 French feeding tube at the breast.

Figure 44. Using a bandage on the breast to hold a supplementer tube in place

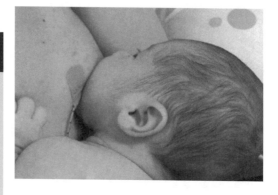

HELPFUL TIPS

MARTA GUÓTH-GUMBERGER, CIVIL ENGINEER AND IBCLC IN GERMANY, RECOMMENDS PLACING THE TUBING ON THE STICKY SIDE OF THE TAPE, AND THEN PLACING THE TAPE AND TUBE ON THE BREAST (GUÓTH-GUMBERGER M., 2006). THIS CAN BE A LESS FRUSTRATING METHOD FOR MOTHERS WHO FEEL THE TUBING "RUNS AWAY" AS THEY TRY TO PIN IT DOWN WITH TAPE.

Smart babies can learn how to just "straw drink" from a supplementer tube. A baby who is straw drinking will have pursed lips and will not use normal jaw excursions. There are several ways to discourage straw drinking, including pulling the tube back a few millimeters so it is slightly behind the tip of the nipple, and re-attaching the baby to ensure a good latch to the breast. If this happens repeatedly, make sure the presence of the tube is not causing the mother to slide the baby's lower lip too close to the nipple during latch. Some mothers concentrate on the baby's upper lip to make sure it clears the tube, and wind up with a shallow attachment, or miss the tube altogether (figure 45). Orienting the tube at the baby's lower lip (figure 46 and 47) can help prevent this difficulty.

Figure 45. Placing the tube at the upper lip may complicate latch.

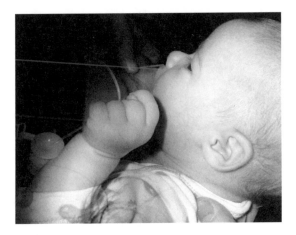

Figure 46. Placing the tube at the lower lip helps obtain a more asymmetrical latch.

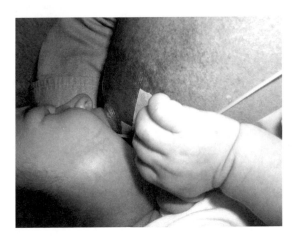

Figure 47. Baby at breast with tube at the lower lip

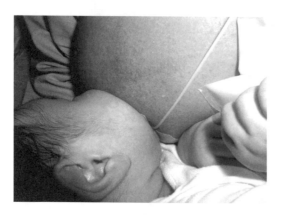

Another potential complication when using a supplementer device is that the baby may grab the device or tubes, or the device may get between mother and baby and interfere with the mother's ability to give the baby stability by holding him close. Setting the supplementer up at the side of the breast rather than between them (figure 48), running the tubing under a nursing bra or tank top (figure 49), or lifting the supplementer higher (figure 50) can all help. With gravity-affected supplementers, such as the SNS or tube in a bottle, the higher the device is in relation to the nipple, the faster the flow will be.

Figure 48. The Lact-Aid can be placed at the side of the breast to keep it out of the way.

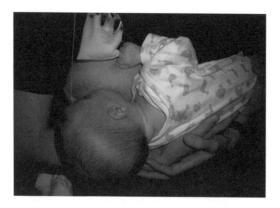

Figure 49. The Lact-Aid is discreet under a nursing top.

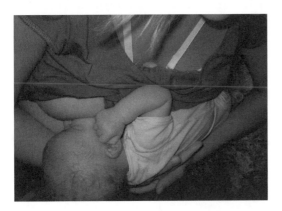

Figure 50. Prevent the SNS from interfering with latch by either lifting it higher on mother's chest or placing it at the side of the breast.

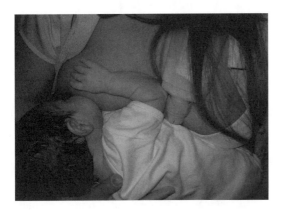

A final issue with choosing between supplementers is the sensory quality of the tubing. Figure 51 illustrates the size and texture differences between some of the feeding tubes.

Figure 51. From left to right: SuppleMate tube; 5 French feeding tube; Lact-Aid tube; SNS tube (largest diameter). Note that all except the Lact-Aid tube are apt to curl.

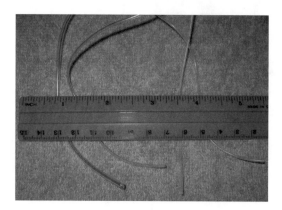

Calculating the Amount of Supplement to Offer

Generally babies are given extra milk when their growth, behavior (unsettledness, crying) or condition (jaundice, dehydration) shows that they have not been transferring sufficient milk. Rarely, the mother has primary lactation insufficiency. More likely, the baby has done a poor job of stimulating her milk production, and the insufficiency is secondary and remediable. In either case, the goal is to provide sufficient milk from the supplementer to achieve good growth and health, without providing so much that less is taken from the breast.

If the baby is in poor condition, giving ad lib supplementation for the first few days can be helpful to restore the baby's energy and ability to work for his feedings (Wilson-Clay & Hoover, 2005). If the growth deficit is smaller or the baby older and more robust, the supplement can be calculated to about 2 ounces per day per ounce of additional weekly weight gain desired. For example, if the baby gained 3 ounces in a week when he should have gained 7, this leaves a deficit of 4 ounces per week. He would need 8 ounces of supplement per day, divided between all or most of his feedings. Since mothers are generally fuller in the morning, the morning feeding, and perhaps middle of the night feedings, can be done without supplementation. For example, the expected weight gain for a male infant under 3 months of age is about 7 ounces per week. A lower weight gain in one week might be due to a temporary illness or inadvertent mismanagement of breastfeeding. However, if there is a pattern of suboptimal growth, documented low milk intake, and breastfeeding management has been improved without improving the baby's growth, supplementation in the following amounts may be needed:

Table 2: Supplementation to Increase Weight Gain

Weight gain (weekly)	6 oz	5 oz	4 oz	3 oz	2 oz	1 oz	zero
Weight deficit (weekly)	1 oz	2 oz	3 oz	4 oz	5 oz	6 oz	7 oz
Supplement amount (daily)	2 oz	4 oz	6 oz	8 oz	10 oz	12 oz	14 oz

The supplementation pattern should be worked out between the LC and the family. If the mother has been feeding the baby for an hour at a time every hour and a half, she is likely to be exhausted. Using a larger bolus of supplement or even giving one large bottle feeding a day as part of the supplement may allow the mother some unbroken sleep to help restore her energy. Sometimes a less than perfect protocol needs to be used in order to sustain the mother's ability to keep breastfeeding. As "Coach" Linda Smith says in her "rules" for lactation consultants, "There's another way" (Smith, 2008). This is a reminder to be flexible in our approach to mothers and to continue searching for solutions if what we've proposed is unacceptable or is not working.

If the infant has difficulty taking additional milk, tolerating the supplement, or still fails to grow well, he should be carefully examined. Unfortunately, health care professionals may be suspicious of breastfeeding itself if there are problems with infant health or growth. Mothers of infants with respiratory, cardiac, or genetic disorders that cause feeding problems or slowed growth have experienced difficulty having their concerns about their infant taken seriously until the infant failed to do better (or did far worse) when supplemented or formula fed. Skilled lactation assessment will usually differentiate a breastfeeding problem from a global problem in the infant (Genna, 2008).

Weaning Off Supplements

If mother is hormonally and anatomically normal, milk production will generally increase within 3-4 days of beginning effective breastfeeding. Production tends to increase slowly at first, then more rapidly as lactocytes (milk making cells) proliferate, mature, and become active. Milk production expands most readily and quickly in the first 6 weeks after the baby's birth, but can be increased at any time during active lactation. Relactation (making milk again after involution) is possible as well, but takes substantially longer. Experienced LCs usually recommend reducing the amount of supplement offered at each feeding by about ½ ounce per feeding every other day. This schedule works best if milk production was not very impaired and mom is healthy and has normally developed breasts that grew during pregnancy or early postpartum. Once the supplement per feeding is down to ½ ounce, the supplement can be discontinued or offered at every other feeding, then every third feeding, until the infant is content with breastfeeding alone. Mothers should expect the infant to breastfeed more frequently at first as supplements are decreased; the increased breastfeeding will help to increase milk production. If the infant is unsettled despite frequent feeding, supplements may need to be increased again, and withdrawn more slowly.

Relactation (making milk after having stopped lactating within the past 6 months) and induced lactation (making milk without a recent pregnancy) proceed more slowly than increasing an "almost sufficient" milk supply. This is due to the need for the milk-making tissue to be built up from a partially or totally involuted state. Some mothers take hormones to simulate the high estrogen, progesterone, and prolactin of pregnancy to help these changes occur, others rely on pumping or breastfeeding with a supplementer to stimulate lactogenesis. Lenore Goldfarb is currently surveying mothers who induced lactation to study the impact of hormonal protocols.

It is important to try to determine the cause of low milk production before counseling the withdrawal of supplements. Mothers with a history of infertility or hormonal imbalances may be at greater risk of intractable low milk production. If hypothyroidism or hyperandrogenism resulted in abnormal breast development during puberty, milk production may remain inadequate even after medical treatment brings hormones to normal levels. Infant growth and satiety should be carefully monitored as a mother with hormonal issues reduces supplements. In situations such as pituitary shock due to postpartum hemorrhage, gestational ovarian theca lutein cyst (Hoover et al., 2002), and maternal diabetes, lactogenesis II may be delayed, but it proceeds normally once it begins. In these cases, weaning from supplements can begin once signs of increasing milk production occur.

Mothers with mild to moderate breast hypoplasia (underdevelopment) may take 6 weeks to increase their milk production to meet infant needs, and if hypoplasia is severe, they may never make sufficient milk (Huggins et al., 2000). For these mothers, the supplement needs to be reduced only after evidence of increased milk production exists, and it needs to be done more slowly and with greater scrutiny of infant growth and satiety. Mothers can be counseled to get weekly or twice weekly weight checks for their infants while supplements are reduced. In high risk situations, an infant scale purchase or rental may be considered.

To Pump or Not To Pump

Ideally, feedings with a supplemental device will be efficient, take 20-30 minutes to complete, and leave time for cleaning the supplementer, as well as pumping to increase milk removal from the breast. If the supplement used is manufactured milk (formula), gastric emptying will be delayed, and feedings will be artificially far apart. Mothers can be advised to express milk midway between feedings or about 45-60 minutes after feeding at least several times a day to help increase breast emptying. In other mammals studied, increased milking frequency in early lactation increases proliferation of milk gland cells and milk production for the balance of lactation (Capuco et al., 2003). Jane Morton, MD, verified that the addition of manual expression to breastfeeding or pumping in the first days after giving birth increases milk production in human mothers as well. A video of Dr. Morton's technique is viewable at http://newborns.stanford.edu/Breastfeeding/ MaxProduction.html Pumping or manual expression may be more than the mother can handle when her baby is difficult to feed. If the mother is unable to express milk, it is very important to ensure that the baby is draining the breast well with the supplementer in place by test weighing (page 109). Generally, the more often and the more fully the breast is drained, the greater the increase in milk production.

Psychological Effects of Supplementers

The emotions of mothers with low milk production are complex, and the supplementer is a physical reminder of mother's production deficit or the baby's feeding difficulties. Mothers may need to express grief and have emotional support for mourning their perfect breastfeeding experience before they are able to move on and use a supplementer. Borucki (2005) found in her naturalistic study of mother's experiences using supplemental feeding tube devices that mothers often had derogatory nicknames for the devices. One of the four major themes identified in this study was "meeting the challenges of the device...The SFTD [Supplemental Feeding Tube Device] was an acceptable alternative that allowed mothers to nourish their infants while meeting their own breastfeeding goals" (p. 431). "Consistently, the mothers spoke about the support of others as being influential in how they managed the challenges of the device" (p. 432). This support took the form of instructions and tips for using the device, practical assistance in using it, and psychosocial support for their efforts to breastfeed despite the frustrations and difficulties of using a supplementer.

There is a high dropout rate in clinical practice in dyads using supplementers. It is important to discuss the challenges inherent in using a supplementer with mothers during the consultation, stressing that if the supplementer seems too overwhelming after a few practice uses, other techniques are available. "This is a starting point, but if this does not work well, there's always a plan B" is one possible way of expressing this. Allowing plenty of time during the consultation for demonstration and return demonstration not only of supplementer use at breast, but of cleaning, assembling, and filling it will help increase the mother's confidence when she is alone with the device.

Alternatives to Supplementers

If maternal milk production is not too reduced, breast compression may increase milk flow to the infant and allow sufficient milk transfer for good growth. In cases where poor breastfeeding management led to insufficient weight gain, a one to two day trial of frequent feeding with good attachment to the breast and breast compression may be reasonable if the infant's energy level is still normal. Underfed newborns quickly lose the energy needed to do the work of feeding and require calories by a practicable method while the mother continues to stimulate her milk production and offer the breast.

If the mother rejects the idea of a supplementer or finds it too difficult, there are several alternatives. One alternative is to feed the required supplement first, then give the breast for "dessert." Another alternative is to pump the breast after feedings. This will help increase milk production and improve the baby's ability to transfer milk. Mothers can reduce supplement given by bottle, cup, finger feeding, or spoon gradually as milk production and baby's feeding skills improve.

Another alternative to a supplementer when the baby is reluctant to breastfeed is the *drip and drop* technique. A spoon or eyedropper can be used to drip milk along the nipple to encourage the baby to attach. While this technique is useful to encourage the baby to attempt breastfeeding, it is not as useful if there is little reward once the baby attaches. Mothers can be taught to express drops of milk onto the nipple to entice a reluctant baby.

Specific Supplementer Devices

Curved Tip Syringe

Figure 52. Curved tip (periodontal) syringe

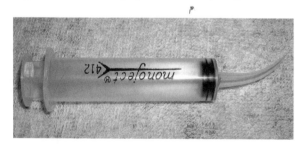

Also called periodontal syringes, curved tip syringes (figure 52) are designed to irrigate the mouth. They are also popular with hobbyists, such as model-makers, for precise placement of glues and resins. This precise control of flow makes them good for supplementing at breast or fingerfeeding, particularly during the first few days of life when milk volume and the infant's needs are low.

Curved tip syringes (Kendall Monoject 412) can be purchased from medical and surgical supply firms, and from veterinary supply companies as well, for about $25 for a box of 50 syringes. Some states do not allow sale of syringes, even syringes that cannot accommodate a needle, to non-physicians. Ordering from a veterinary supply company avoids this issue, and the syringes are identical to those from medical supply firms.

Use

Latch the infant onto the breast and then slip the syringe tip into the corner of the mouth. Maintain gentle pressure against the breast to avoid pressing the rigid syringe tip against the baby's lips or tongue. As the baby sucks, deliver small boluses by gently pressing the plunger. Stop delivering milk as needed to allow normal respiratory pauses.

Price

$25 for a box of 50 syringes

Contact Information

Many medical and veterinary supply houses, including http://www. atozvetsupply.com/Monoject-Curved-Tip-Syringe-50-ct-p/10-mj-ct.htm

Advantages

- Provides excellent control over milk delivery, including flow rate, timing of flow, and bolus size
- Very inexpensive (50 cents each in box of 50)

Disadvantages

- Sales to non-physicians may be restricted in some states
- Small capacity (12cc)
- Perceived as sharp, may worry parents
- May require awkward hand position to use
- Rubber gasket on plunger breaks down when exposed to detergent (washing with bar soap extends life)

Suggested Uses

- Use as treatment probe during consultation (is the supplementing at breast technique useful for this infant?)
- Can be used to pre-fill shield teat for an instant reward for infants who are reluctant to latch (figure 28) as it fits in holes in nipple shield teat
- Can be used to aim a squirt of milk at mom's nipple as baby approaches, to reward attempts at latching and direct baby's efforts

- Can be used to supplement an infant with cleft palate at breast (It allows milk to be aimed onto the tongue and away from the cleft. Milk should be supplied in small boluses in synchrony with the infants sucking efforts.)

Tube and Syringe

A feeding or blood collection tube and syringe can also be used to supplement an infant at breast. Different sizes and types of tubes can be used on a syringe to provide additional milk as the baby sucks. Butterfly tubing is soft and has a luer lock female connector at one end and a needle with silicone wings for stabilization at the other end. The needle should be cut off with clean or sterile scissors before use as a feeding tube as shown in figure 53.

Figure 53. Blood collection tubes can be used for at-breast supplementation if the needle is removed.

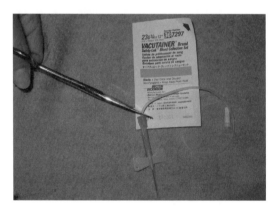

Figure 54. A 5 French feeding tube with a luer slip connector on a luer slip tip syringe

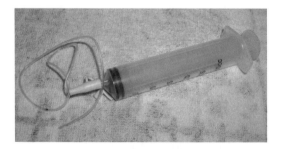

Feeding tubes (figure 54) are generally made of polyvinylchloride (PVC) and have a sealed, rounded tip and two ports (holes), one at either side of the tube a few mm behind the tip. This arrangement of holes releases milk laterally, not straight out the front of the tube like an open tube would. Some practitioners cut off the tip of the feeding tube to avoid loss of milk if the tube is not sufficiently far enough in the mouth to enclose both holes. If the port end is cut off, the LC should cut straight across the tube to avoid leaving a beveled edge with a sharp point. 5 French tubes are generally used, as this size is traditionally used for feeding preterm infants. A newer silicone feeding tube is also available that is slightly less stiff, has a smooth rounded tip, and has a smaller port in the tip, as well as the traditional two at the sides. Tubes come in various lengths from shorter 9 and 12 inch to 36 inch. Hospital based LCs tend to use the shorter lengths, as these are usually available in the nursery, and a shorter tube avoids losing precious colostrum in the tubing. Private practice LCs tend to use longer tubing to give mothers more freedom of hand placement. The opposite end of the tube generally has a luer female connector that mates with a luer lock or luer slip syringe, but some come with a catheter connector (particularly those sold for veterinary use). It is necessary to use the correct syringe to mate with the tube's connector.

A syringe filled with milk is attached to the connector, and the tube is placed or taped at the breast so that the tube is grasped by the baby's tongue along with the breast when the baby attaches (Benakappa, 2002). Benakappa also recommends taping over the proximal (farther from the tip) port in the tube, and taping the tube along the breast and up to the clavicle before attaching the syringe.

Luer lock syringes have a short plastic sleeve around the inner connector to avoid the tube being dislodged. Luer slip syringes have a longer male connector with no outer sleeve The slip tip can be at the center of the syringe, or it can be offset toward the periphery, in which case it's called an eccentric tip. Luer slip eccentric tip syringes are especially useful for drawing up smaller volumes of human milk from the edges of a pump container or bottle. See figure 55 for a comparison of these different syringe types.

Figure 55. Left: Luer lock syringe, note the threads; Center: Luer slip eccentric tip; Right: Luer slip tip

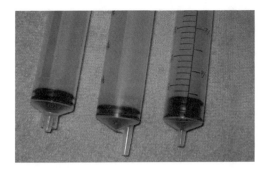

The volume of the syringe to be used depends on the volume needs of the infant and the hand size of the mother. A small 3 or 10 ml syringe is ideal in the first few days postpartum when volumes of colostrum are smaller. Using a smaller syringe in the first 2 days postpartum reinforces appropriate expectations for milk production in new mothers. After day 3 or so as infant needs increase, a 30 to 35 ml syringe usually is ideal as it is large enough to fit a significant proportion of the infant's supplement, while being small enough for the mother to use comfortably. When milk volume is small, it's best to draw up the milk into the syringe by placing the tip of the syringe in the milk and pulling back on the plunger. When there is greater milk volume, the LC can decide whether it is better to use the syringe intact or to pull out the plunger and pour the milk into the back of the syringe barrel. Using the syringe with the plunger allows the adult to help bolus the baby. This is advantageous when the baby has lost significant weight and has low energy. The LC needs to carefully instruct the mother to synchronize her bolus with the baby's sucking efforts so she is supporting the baby's coordination of swallowing and breathing. Providing flow when the baby needs a respiratory break can cause hypoxia by suppressing breathing or provoke aspiration if the baby tries to breathe with fluid in the airway. Taking the time during the consultation to have the parent return demonstrate the technique is vital to avoiding these problems. Figure 56 shows a mother feeding her infant at breast with a 5 French feeding tube on a syringe.

Figure 56. Using a feeding tube and syringe to supplement at the breast. The breast pump is not turned on, it is being used to catch milk dripping from the contralateral breast.

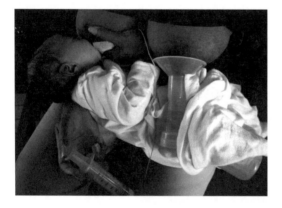

There are several challenges for the mother using a syringe with a plunger. One challenge is having a hand free to hold the syringe while supporting her baby at breast. Using an ergonomic breastfeeding position so most of the baby's weight is on the mother's trunk and not on her arms as shown in figure 57 can address this issue. Another challenge is having the hand strength needed to depress the plunger.

Repetitive stress injuries, such as carpal tunnel syndrome, are common during pregnancy and impact a mother's ability to push the plunger. Keeping the wrist neutral (neither flexed toward the body or extended away) reduces wrist pain and strain. If mom lacks hand strength, she can upend the syringe and push the syringe onto the plunger while it rests on her thigh or another handy surface as in figure 58.

Figure 57. If mother reclines and keeps baby at her nipple's natural height, she can spare a hand to use the syringe.

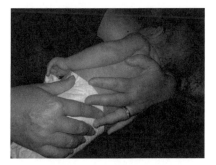

Figure 58. This mother is using an ergonomic breastfeeding position where gravity helps support her infant. She is pressing the syringe plunger against her thigh to avoid hand strain.

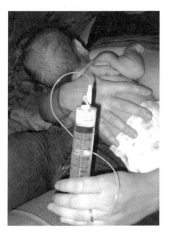

There are also challenges to overcome if the syringe is used without the plunger. There is no pressure holding the milk in the syringe when the plunger is removed, so it flows much more freely. The higher the syringe is held, the faster the flow will be because of acceleration due to gravity. It is easy to spill the open syringe. Some mothers rest the syringe in their cleavage, particularly if they are wearing a bra, others tape it to their chest above or between the breasts with first aid tape. Some mothers latch the baby on to the breast and tube, and then fill the syringe while it is taped to their body or snuggled in their bra to avoid losing milk. Mothers who are athletic and coordinated or who have previously breastfed an infant are more likely to be able to successfully use this technique than mothers who are inexperienced with breastfeeding and more likely to need all their attention to give their infants support at the breast.

Use

Draw milk into the syringe and attach a feeding tube. The tube can be taped to the breast and the infant latched, or slipped into the corner of the baby's mouth after he is fixed to the breast. As the baby sucks, press the plunger gently and slowly to deliver small quantities of milk (less than 1 ml per suck). Make sure to stop delivering milk when the baby stops for respiratory pauses. If the infant does not pause as needed and shows signs of stress, such as finger-splaying, a distressed expression, or loud swallowing, stop the flow for at least 3-5 seconds, or until the baby's respiratory rate returns to baseline. Particularly competent infants may be able to move milk from the syringe with the plunger in place, and will not require bolusing.

Price

$70 for a case of 50 tubes from Grogan's (5 French, 36 inch length); up to $4 each in retail surgical supply stores

Contact Information

http://www.grogans.com/servlet/shop?cmd=I&id=KEN155721

Advantages

- Adult can pace the feeding, can provide boluses to keep baby sucking
- Adult can supplement baby's efforts, giving more food for less work
- Readily available materials
- Inexpensive

Disadvantages

- Some states restrict syringe sales physicians only
- Some risk management attorneys forbid non-standard use of materials in a hospital setting. Others are not concerned as feeding tubes are designed for infant feeding and are designed to be used with syringes.

- Medical equipment can frighten some parents. This may be visceral and difficult to change, or discussion may allow reframing and increased parental comfort.

- Rigid tubing can deform infant's palate if repeatedly placed between the breast and palate.

- Syringe can be painful to use if mother has carpal tunnel syndrome or other hand conditions.

Suggested Uses

- Short term use when baby has lost significant weight. Mom can provide bolus when baby sucks, and allow appropriate respiratory breaks. This often keeps a baby who has low energy reserves feeding for longer to allow recovery and catch-up growth.

- Short term use for mother to decide if supplementing at breast is a viable option before purchasing a more expensive device

- For mothers who are overwhelmed easily, the syringe and tube might be suitable because of their ease of assembly, use, and cleaning.

- Can be used to supplement an infant with a cleft palate who is unable to produce negative intraoral pressure at breast (Boluses should be small, and timed in concert with the infant's sucking efforts. The tube should be placed between the breast and the tongue to avoid milk entering the cleft. Straddle or prone positioning at breast may help reduce entry of milk into the cleft as well.)

- Can be used as the first step in using multiple supplementers to help an infant develop correct negative intraoral pressure. At first, the mother depresses the syringe. Once the baby is noted to attempt to make negative pressure (pulling milk out of the syringe by himself or more normal suction felt at breast), a more challenging supplementer, such as a tube in a bottle (Dr. Jack Newman's Lactation Aid) or a commercial device, can be tried. This multiple supplementer technique can be useful in infants whose sucking skills preclude the immediate use of a supplementer that requires competence. Examples include infants who do not spontaneously suck well after frenotomy, preterm infants who are not producing negative pressure well, and infants with soft palate dysfunction.)

SuppleMate™

Figure 59. Maternal Concepts® SuppleMate™ Infant Care I

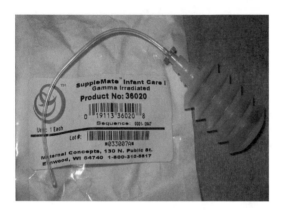

This small, temporary use supplementer (pictured in figure 59) consists of a one ounce plastic accordion pleated reservoir with a narrow neck into which a plug and tubing unit inserts. The tubing is short and stiff, comparable in diameter to an 8 French feeding tube. They are sterile packed and ready to use as is, requiring no additional parts. The easiest way to fill the container is to compress it bottom to top, insert the end of the tube into the milk, let go, and allow the container to draw in the milk as it resumes its shape. If the tube is removed, the container can also be filled with a syringe or with a narrow funnel. The tube can be slipped into the corner of the baby's mouth while at the breast or held or taped near the nipple while baby attaches. The container is sufficiently soft that the baby can draw the milk with negative pressure, or the feeder can bolus the baby. Boluses tend to be large as a small press moves a lot of milk due to the diameter of the container in relation to its volume. Rinsing is as simple as sucking up soapy and then clear water and pushing them out through the tube. The plug can be removed for cleaning around the rim of the container. Thorough cleaning is difficult if milk is allowed to dry inside, both due to the narrow neck and the folds of the container. The SuppleMate I has a 6 inch tube and is designed for supplementing at the breast. The SuppleMate Infant Care II has a 2 inch tube and is designed for fingerfeeding.

Use

Slip the tube into the infant's mouth after latching, or hold to breast while latching infant. If the baby does not suck effectively, press the bottom of the container gently to deliver milk. Ensure the infant stops for respiratory pauses, or impose them by stopping the flow.

Price

$3.50 each, bulk prices available ($2.00 each for 100 units)

Contact Information

Maternal Concepts http://www.maternalconcepts.com/

1.800.310.5817

Advantages

- Inexpensive
- Self-contained, nothing else needed.
- Sterile packed, pre-assembled
- Easy to use, requires only one hand, can also be picked up and used after baby is latched.
- Stable when placed on its bottom, keeps the tube upright and away from potentially contaminated surfaces.

Disadvantages

- Very stiff tubing, difficult to use with nipple shield
- May distort palate with frequent use if placed between breast and baby's palate
- Designed for short term use - pleated container can crack with repeated use, difficult to clean thoroughly

Suggested Uses

- Ideal for in hospital supplementation of newborns, as it is designed for supplementing at breast, sterile packed, inexpensive, requires no extra parts, and holds a realistic feeding volume for infants under 72 hours old. The SuppleMate is also useful as a "treatment probe" to see if supplementing at breast produces the desired results before the mother invests in a more expensive and more permanent device.

Tube in a Bottle (Lactation Aid)

Figure 60. Home-assembled Lactation Aid

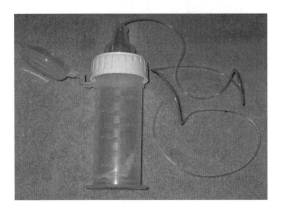

Dr. Jack Newman popularized the use of a 5 French feeding tube in a bottle of milk to assist an infant having difficulty breastfeeding or a mother with low milk production. The luer connector end of the tube is placed in a bottle, and the port end is threaded through a bottle nipple, with the hole enlarged to a slit with a knife or scissors, from the inside to the outside (figure 60). After assuring that the luer end of the tube is at the bottom of the bottle, the nipple is screwed on to prevent leaking. The bottle is placed in mom's cleavage or on furniture next to her. The longer the tube, the longer the infant has to suck before he draws milk from the tube. A shorter tube can be helpful if the infant is reluctant to breastfeed because the rewarding milk flows to the baby more quickly. Milk flow rate can be increased by lifting the bottle higher so the milk flows downward with gravity. As the baby becomes more secure that he will get milk at the breast, it can be helpful to use a longer tube or to place the bottle lower to simulate sucking until the Milk Ejection Reflex occurs. Figure 61 illustrates one way to set up this device for a reluctant breastfeeder – the tube is short and the bottle is placed in mother's cleavage to maximize flow.

As the baby becomes more skillful at breastfeeding, the mother can gradually increase the length of the tubing, and place the bottle lower to decrease the milk flow from the tubing, perhaps on a pile of telephone books or a stool on the floor. As with any supplementer device, providing a flow that leads to effective sucking (a 1:1:1 to 2:1:1 suck:swallow:breathe ratio during active sucking, if the infant's aerobic capacity allows) (Genna, 2008) is the goal.

Unless the feeding tube is to be replaced for every feeding, it is wise to provide a syringe for cleaning the inside of the tubing. The outside can be cleaned by soaking in soapy water or washing with a clean, soapy sponge and rinsing. To clean the inside of the tube, draw a few cc's of soapy water into the syringe, push them out through the tube, rinse the syringe, and then push clear water through the tubing to rinse out the soap. Pushing air through the tubing will push out any residual water and reduce the chance of mineral scale forming.

Figure 61. Repurposing a fast flow nipple into a lactation aid. Note the modified adhesive bandage to hold the tube in place.

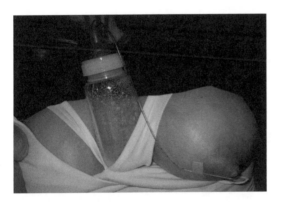

Use

Tape the feeding tube to the breast or slip into the corner of the infant's mouth after latching. Raise the bottle high to start milk flow. Once the infant begins receiving supplement, lower the bottle slightly until the best suck:swallow:breathe rhythm possible is achieved. Allow the infant to pace the feeding. If the baby becomes discouraged, raise the bottle to increase the ease of flow again.

Price

Depends on the price of the components. Feeding tubes range from $1.50 to $4.00, depending on place of purchase; bottles can cost less than $1 including nipple unit, or up to $10 each if certified BPA free. A Snappies container with a hole drilled in the lid and a feeding tube both purchased in bulk will cost less than $2.

Contact Information

See Snappies (page 153) and Tube and Syringe (page 78).

Advantages

- Inexpensive
- Simple to assemble and clean
- Effective
- Provides a use for inappropriately fast flowing bottle nipples

Disadvantages

- Difficult to use discreetly (If mom wants to hide the bottle in her bra under her shirt, a narrow bottle, such as a 70 cc Snappies, can be used.)

- Need to make sure the end of the tubing stays submerged in the milk

Suggested Uses

- Works well when mom has reduced milk production and a reasonably competent baby. A method that allows easier provision of boluses may be better if the infant is sleepy, has low energy reserves, or is reluctant to breastfeed. If mom can support the infant with one hand, she can use the other hand to raise the bottle higher and increase the flow from the tube temporarily until the baby generates a good sucking rhythm.

Figure 62. Eliminating the need for a nipple by making a hole in a bottle sealing disk. Photo courtesy of Kay Hoover, IBCLC.

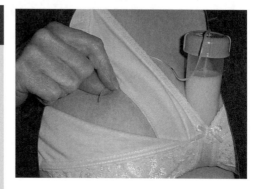

HELPFUL TIPS

KAY HOOVER PUTS THE HOLE NEARER THE BASE OF THE NIPPLE TO MAKE INSERTING THE TUBE EASIER, OR USES A DRILL WITH A FINE BIT TO DRILL A HOLE IN THE SEALING DISK OF THE BOTTLE TO ELIMINATE THE NEED FOR A NIPPLE. FIGURES 62 AND 63 ILLUSTRATE THESE MODIFICATIONS.

Figure 63. Making a hole at the base of the nipple makes it easier to feed the tube through the nipple. Photo courtesy of Kay Hoover, IBCLC.

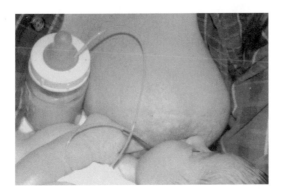

If mom doesn't have a bottle, any clean container will work. I've used sterile urine specimen containers. They are a good size, are stable and unlikely to tip over, are sterile, and the thin plastic cover is easy to pierce with a fork or knife to make a hole for the tubing.

Sneak Peek: Ameda Supplemental Feeding System

Figure 64. Prototype Ameda Supplemental Feeding System

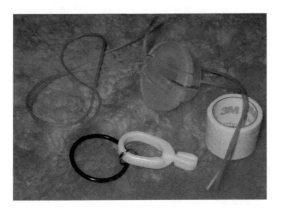

Figure 65. Ameda Supplemental Feeding System assembled, using a Snappies breastmilk container.

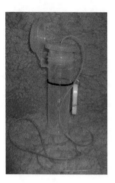

Ameda is developing an inexpensive lactation aid kit inspired by Dr. Newman (figures 64 and 65). The main feature is a plastic plug that fits into standard bottles to hold one or two thin, flexible sterile tubes. The plug is split for easy insertion of the tubes. The pre-sterilized kit will come with several tubes, the bottle plug, a rubber ring and clothing clip, and a small roll of paper first-aid tape. Refill supplies of sterile tubing will be available separately, as the tubing is not easily washable. The tubing will likely be long enough that each tube can be cut in half if desired. Flow dynamics will likely be very similar to using a 5 French feeding tube in a bottle. My prototype is not cleared for human use, so I was not able to use it with infants. It seems like it will be a good addition to the tool kit - a sterile, inexpensive, ready-to-use nursing supplementer with replaceable tubing. The need to use a new piece of tubing for each feeding is less than kind to the environment, but increases the safety of use for ill or preterm infants.

Starter SNS™

Figure 66. Medela Starter SNS

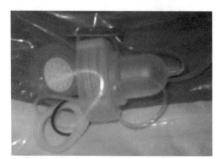

The Starter Supplemental Nursing System™ (figure 66) is a temporary ready-to-use supplementer device. It comes sterile, with or without a container, and is designed to be used for 24 hours. The tube is short and comes with a notched plastic piece to close off flow. The threads fit standard bottles, Snappies and VoluFeeds. The black elastic band with the clothing clip is placed around the bottle, the bottle is filled with supplement, and the Starter SNS is screwed on. The device is "primed" by squeezing the reservoir while the tube is upright, then inverting it and releasing to allow some milk to enter the bulb. The tubing is then crimped off, and the clothing clip is attached to the mother's clothing.

Cleaning

The tubing is cleaned by assembling the device with soapy water in the container, inverting it, and squeezing the reservoir. This is repeated with clear water until no soap residue remains in the tubing.

Use

Assemble and clip to clothing. Tape tube to the breast with the tape included in the packaging, or hold to breast while latching baby. Open the tubing to allow milk to flow. If the baby struggles with the flow, move the container lower on the body or crimp the tubing to allow a breathing break. Once the feeding is over, discard any milk in the reservoir. Clean carefully with soapy water, forcing water through the tubes by pressing on the reservoir. Repeat with clean water to rinse. Discard after 24 hours, especially if used with manufactured baby milk.

Price

$8-9

Contact Information

Medela, Inc. http://www.medelabreastfeedingus.com/

1.800.435.8316

Advantages

- Prepackaged for hospital use

Disadvantages

- Expensive for manufacturers suggested life of 24 hours
- Any milk that enters the reservoir needs to be evacuated through the tube and will be wasted if not consumed by the infant.
- Clothing clip is cumbersome and doesn't always hold well, some LCs substitute a large safety pin (diaper pin).
- Difficult to use if mother is not wearing a shirt or bra, as it lacks a neck strap.

Suggested Use

- Short term use in an environment where other alternatives are unacceptable, such as when the risk-management team discourages the use of a syringe and tube

- Short term use when a thin soft tube is particularly useful (as for a baby with a strong gag reflex).

Lact-Aid® Nursing Trainer

Figure 67. The Lact-Aid® is useful for low milk production.

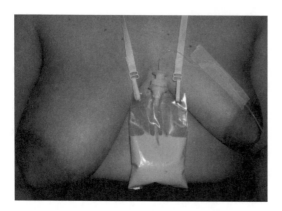

Figure 68. The Lact-Aid® tubing can also be taped along the breast where the baby's lower lip will land. Slipping the tube under the mother's clothing helps keep it in place and prevents the baby from pulling on it.

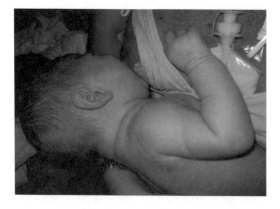

Figure 69. Milk flows through the Lact-Aid® tubing when the baby's posterior tongue and jaw move downward, the same movement that removes milk from the breast.

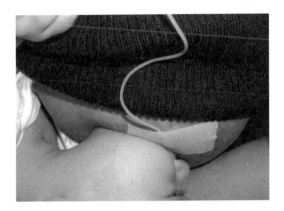

The Lact-Aid® was designed for use by mothers with extremely low milk production, as in adoptive breastfeeding or relactation. It consists of a tubing unit that secures into a specially designed sterile plastic bag to hold the supplement, which is held around the neck with a modified lingerie strap. It is easy to assemble with a little practice, can be pre-filled and refrigerated, and is easily heated as the plastic bag transmits heat readily. The tube is relatively short, making it easier to keep out of the infant's reach. When air is evacuated from the device during assembly as per the instructions, supplement flows rapidly to give the infant a reward for sucking, but it does not readily leak (figure 67). Mothers with pendulous breasts may have difficulty getting the tube in the right place without extending the necklace, or removing one side and hooking it around the bra. The mother in figure 68 has removed one end of the strap and is allowing the Lact-Aid to sit in her nursing tank top. Accessories that make it more pleasant to use are available, such as a pretty white eyelet holder that secures to the neck strap or bra. Bags are available in 4 ounce and 7 ounce capacities, but use of the 7 ounce bags requires an extension kit for the tubing unit.

The use of the Lact-Aid during breastfeeding was shown to be effective in increasing milk production and infant growth (when used with and without prolactin stimulating medications) in a case series (Weichert, 1980), although the mechanism of action proposed (replenishing prolactin in the brain by reducing the frequency of feeding) has been invalidated by subsequent research. In actuality, milk flows from the bag when the infant uses negative pressure sucking (figure 69), eliminating the cycle of constantly feeding, but getting little milk that can occur when mothers have low milk production. The faster milk flow keeps most infants sucking more diligently and improves breast drainage accordingly.

Assembly of the Lact-Aid can feel intimidating to the new LC. Each Lact-Aid kit contains an illustrated step-by-step instruction guide, similar to the "quick start guides" that come with computer hardware. The basic steps are simple:

- tear a bag off the roll at the perforations (figure 70),

- remove the perforated tabs on either side of the spout or neck of the bag,

- place the bag upright in a cup or mug for easy filling, rub with fingers to open (figure 71),

- place the funnel in the neck of the bag and fill with milk (figure 72) (if desired, use the bracket to hold the bag, figure 73),

- if using powdered formula, strain out lumps by placing the included strainer in the funnel before filling,

- remove the funnel, and place the wider end of the tubing unit in the neck of the bag, up to the white plug connecting the wider and narrower tubing (figure 74),

- separate the ring-shaped collar (sealing ring) from the tubing unit and place it over the neck of the bag (figure 75),

- continue to push the white plug downward until it fits snugly into the neck of the bag (figure 76),

- lift the sealing ring (collar) to seal the bag against the plug (figure 77).

It's wise to check the seal by lifting the unit an inch or two by the plug end. If the seal is not tight, the bag will fall back into the cup, and the milk will be preserved. After the seal is checked, air can be evacuated by turning the unit upside down, so the wide tube is in the air pocket, and gently squeezing the bag. This has the potential to drip some milk from the tube. To preserve any hard-won milk mom has pumped, the air can also be evacuated by gently squeezing the bag just before the plug completely seals the neck. The air does not have to be completely removed for the device to work. To prevent leaking until the device is used, the collar (sealing ring) contains slits to slide the tubing into to pinch off the flow (figure 78).

The manufacturer's instructions recommend disconnecting the two parts of the tubing unit with a hex wrench and cleaning the thinner feeding tube with soapy water through the bottom of the plug, using the supplied bulb syringe (figure 79). The bulb syringe can be held with the tip against the end of the wider end of the tubing and a finger and thumb used to hold the two devices together, directing the water through the entire tubing unit (figure 80). Soapy water is used until the tube is clear, and then a 50% white vinegar and water solution is used to rinse to remove both soap residues and residual milk fat. The manufacturer recommends re-rinsing the unit with distilled water after cleaning to prevent mineral scale from forming in the tubing thereby reducing the flow rate. Using the enclosed bulb syringe to push air through the tubing will similarly reduce mineral scale formation if tap water is used. The air will push out the rinse water, preventing the water from evaporating in the tubing and leaving its' mineral load behind. If mineral scale does form in the tubing, rinsing it and soaking it in equal parts white vinegar and water will help dissolve the scale and restore proper flow.

Figures 70-80. Lact-Aid® Assembly and Cleaning

Figure 70.

Figure 71.

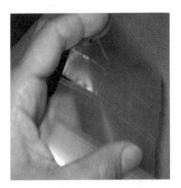
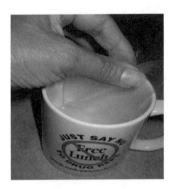

Figure 72.

Figure 73

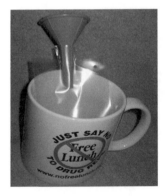
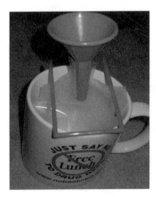

Figure 74.

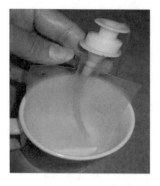

Figure 75.

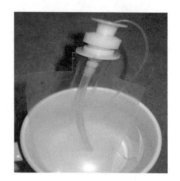

Figure 76.

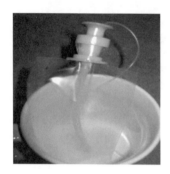

Figure 77.

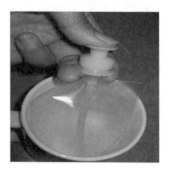

Figure 78.

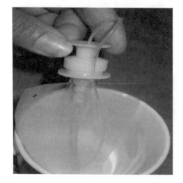

Figure 79.

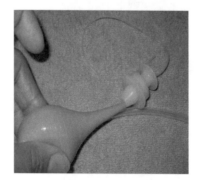

Figure 80.

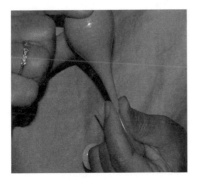

With a little practice, cleaning the tubing and refilling the device takes only a minute or two. The refilled device can be placed in the refrigerator or in a cooler until needed, and used cold or warmed by placing the bag in a cup of warm water if desired. Jimmie Lynn Avery, inventor of Lact-Aid, recommends pre-priming the tubing immediately after filling if the Lact-aid will be stored in the refrigerator before use. This is achieved by upending the device and squeezing it until the thin tubing is full of milk. Pre-priming prevents minerals from the rinse water from sticking in the tubing and reducing flow rates.

If powdered formula is used in the Lact-aid, it should not be stored more than one hour after mixing, as it is not a sterile product and bacterial contamination is common (Labiner-Wolfe et al., 2008). When filling the Lact-aid with powdered formula, the strainer should be placed in the funnel (solid side up) to catch any lumps to prevent them from clogging the tubing. If clogs form anyway, rubbing the tubing between two fingers will help disperse them, and a vinegar rinse after use will dissolve them.

Using the Lact-Aid

The lingerie strap clips are inserted in the holes in the bag, and the unit is placed around the neck. The strap can be shortened to bring the bag to the desired height, a few inches above the nipple is ideal, so that the tube reaches the nipple and can be held or taped in place while the baby latches. The instructions recommend placing the tube at the center of the baby's upper lip, but this can sometimes obstruct latch or fail to get the tube in the mouth (figure 45). The tube can also be placed at the center of baby's lower lip, so it winds up over the baby's tongue (figures 46, 47, and 68). It is more difficult to identify if the baby missed the tube, but if no milk flows from the device when the baby sucks, this is the likely reason. In this case, the baby should be reattached.

Generally, the flow rate from the Lact-Aid is controlled by the baby. If the bag is placed between mother and baby, the baby's weight against the bag will increase the milk flow. Mom can also press on the bag if faster flow is needed. It is important that flow not be pushed beyond that necessary to interest the baby in sucking. Part of the reason that LCs supplement babies at the breast is to reinforce the contingent nature of feeding – that sucking causes milk to flow into the mouth. If milk flow is unpredictable and not tied to the baby's activity, baby has no effective feedback to guide his actions.

Rarely, the narrower tubing crimps or is blocked by a lump from powdered formula or dried milk. Rinsing with a 50% white vinegar and water solution and rubbing the tube between thumb and finger is usually sufficient to release the crimp or clog. The vinegar also helps sanitize the tubing.

Use

Assemble as illustrated above, and hang the Lact-Aid around the neck or pin to the bra. Hold or tape the tube to the breast and allow the baby to attach. Release the tubing from the pinch point in the sealing ring, and breastfeed as usual. Can also be used in sidelying positions, as gravity is not needed for flow.

Price

$28 wholesale in quantities of 12 or more, $50 retail

Contact Information

Lact-Aid International   www.Lact-Aid.com

1.866.866.1239

Advantages

- Higher maternal satisfaction than other supplementers – participants of the BFAR (Breastfeeding After Breast Reduction) e-group who have used multiple commercial supplementers were more likely to prefer the Lact-Aid than other devices. In my own practice, I've found that many mothers dislike the Lact-Aid less than other supplementer devices, though I carry and use all of them (commercial and home-made).

- Still manufactured and sold by the couple who invented it: Jimmie Lynne Avery promptly answers callers with questions or concerns.

- Very discreet under clothing

- Effective

Disadvantages

- More complicated to assemble than a syringe and tube or bottle and tube.

HELPFUL TIPS

MODIFICATION FOR CLEFT AFFECTED INFANTS - THE LACT AID INNER TUBE (BAG TUBE) CAN BE SCREWED OFF AND THE DEVICE ASSEMBLED AND TURNED UPSIDE DOWN TO PROVIDE FLOW WITHOUT NEGATIVE PRESSURE AS ILLUSTRATED IN FIGURE 81. MOM CONTROLS THE FLOW BY COMPRESSING AND RELEASING THE TUBE IN CONCERT WITH THE BABY'S SUCKING. SHE RELEASES THE TUBE WHEN THE BABY SUCKS, THEN COMPRESSES IT TO PREVENT MILK FLOW, WHILE THE BABY SWALLOWS AND BREATHES, RELEASING IT BRIEFLY FOR THE NEXT SUCK. WHILE CAREFUL TEACHING IS IMPORTANT TO PREVENT THE BABY FROM BEING OVERWHELMED WITH FLOW, MOTHERS LEARN THEIR INFANT'S RHYTHMS WITH A LITTLE PRACTICE. THIS TECHNIQUE IS CERTAINLY NO MORE RISKY THAN FEEDING WITH A TRADITIONAL SQUEEZE BOTTLE (MEAD JOHNSON CLEFT PALATE FEEDER). THE INFANT IS UNLIKELY TO REMOVE MUCH MILK FROM THE BREAST (THE MOTHER WILL NEED TO EXPRESS TO FILL THE LACT-AID), BUT FEEDING AT BREAST KEEPS THE BABY'S FEEDING BREAST-FOCUSED, SO THAT WHEN THE CLEFT IS REPAIRED, THE INFANT WILL BREASTFEED. BREASTFEEDING IS ALSO LIKELY TO HELP NORMALIZE TONGUE FUNCTION, WHICH CAN BE PROBLEMATIC FOR CLEFT-AFFECTED BABIES.

- Waste and cost of disposable bags (though this is balanced by less water and polluting detergents needed for cleaning)

- Needs to be washed before first use

- Requires a fairly competent baby, capable of generating negative pressure.

Suggested Uses

- Experienced clinicians feel that this device is the most effective supplementer to use when maternal milk production is low. The lack of gravity effects, reliable flow, and need for baby to use negative intraoral pressure (normal breastfeeding sucking) to move milk from the device all help pattern good feeding behaviors while nourishing the baby. Demonstrating the cleaning, assembly, and filling; talking the mother through her return demonstration; and then staying while she cleans and re-fills the device at the end of the consultation will increase her confidence.

When long term supplementation will be needed for a baby with a normal or near normal ability to create intraoral negative pressure, the Lact-Aid is a good choice. Since there is no rigid container and additional tubing units are available for sale, mothers can continue an active lifestyle and just take several filled units with them in a small cooler. The Lact-Aid can be slipped underneath mom's shirt through the neck band, and the baby breastfed without exposing the device, especially when the tube is placed at the baby's lower lip.

Weaning off the Lact-Aid

Weaning can occur naturally: as the breast increases production, the flow rate from the breast increases, and the baby's mouth fills mostly with milk from the breast, so less is taken from the Lact-Aid. Once the breast begins to respond to the improved sucking stimulus (generally 3-4 days after supplementation was begun, but this may vary and requires assessment by the lactation consultant), the amount of supplement can be gradually decreased. Many practitioners find that reducing the amount of milk in the Lact-Aid by ½ ounce per feeding every other day is a good rate for mothers with normal breasts and normal hormonal status. Periodic assessment of infant intake from the breast by test weights of the infant and the Lact-Aid before and after feeding can inform the speed of supplement reduction. The mother can also be guided by infant behavior and growth. If the baby is content after feeding and continues to grow at expected rates, all is well. A weekly weight check at the infant's doctor's office or the Lactation Consultant's office may be recommended during weaning from supplements.

Once supplement is down to ½ to 1 ounce per feeding, the LC may wish to recommend using the device at fewer feedings. Many babies seem content after their first morning breastfeed without a supplementer, and others are happy to breastfeed at night in bed with mother without the device. Mothers can be advised to stop using the device at these feedings first, and then start alternating feedings with and without the Lact-Aid. After a day or two, another feeding can be done without the supplementer and the baby's behavior and growth monitored. If the baby is fussy and does not settle when offered the breast alone, supplementer use can be increased.

Figure 81. Lact-aid modification for use with cleft affected infants

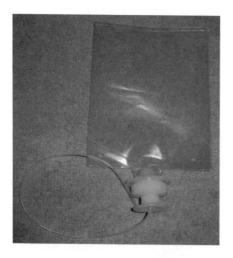

Medela Supplemental Nursing System™ (SNS)

Figure 82. Medela SNS™

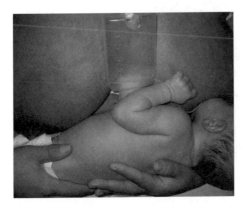

The Supplemental Nursing System™ (SNS)(figure 82), manufactured by Medela, consists of a rigid plastic container with a narrow mouth that accommodates twin tubes attached to venting "valves." The cap assembly can be fussy: the valve membrane needs to be completely dry and sit absolutely flat on the valve cover in order to avoid leakage. Three different diameters of tubing are included, giving this system flexibility in flow characteristics. It is the most complex supplementer to use, as there are many variables that affect flow – height of the container, size of the tubing, and whether the opposite tube is left crimped or is open to vent the container as shown in figure 83. If the LC is savvy to all the variables and the client good with details, the SNS can be a flexible system and can help meet the baby's need for supplement flow rate. However, many LCs just use the medium tubing, place the supplementer cap at nipple height, and crimp the unused tube. Bolusing is possible, but the container is rather rigid and takes some hand strength to squeeze.

Figure 83. Using the SNS with one tube vented to reduce resistance to flow

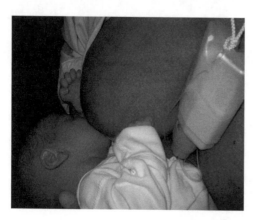

Modifying Flow

To increase flow, raise container above nipple height, use wider tubing, vent the unused tube by leaving it open and taping it to side of the SNS container (pointing upward to avoid leaking) (figure 83).

To decrease flow, lower container cap below nipple height, use narrower tubing, and pinch off the unused tube.

Especially when hung high with the largest tubing, the SNS seems to provide a freer flow with less negative pressure exerted by the baby. This can be helpful if the infant has soft palate dysfunction and is unable to fully seal the back of the oral cavity. It can also be helpful in cases of relactation where maternal milk production is very low and a higher milk flow is needed to keep the baby interested at breast. The SNS used at maximum flow may also be helpful for supplementing infants who have reduced energy for feeding, but do have normal respiratory capacities.

If the SNS tubes have been wrapped in a tight circle, they tend to retain some curvature. This can cause the tube to stick out and make latching to both the tube and the breast difficult. If any curve in the end of the tube is oriented toward the nipple, the tube is less likely to bend away from the breast. The current packaging avoids tightly coiling the tube, but the instructions advise protecting the tubing by wrapping it around the inside of the cap before putting the cover on for travel.

Assembly

Figures 84 through 91. SNS Assembly

Figure 84.   **Figure 85.**

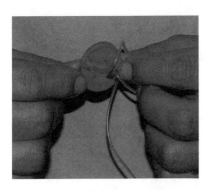 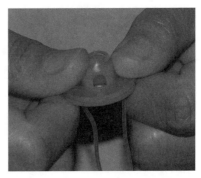

Figure 86.   **Figure 87.**

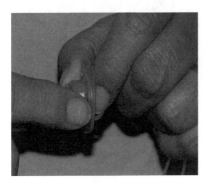 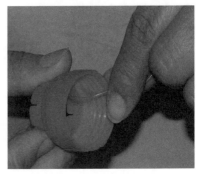

Figure 88.   **Figure 89.**

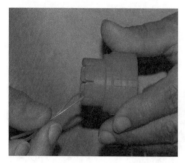
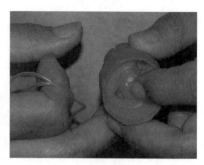

Figure 90.   **Figure 91.**

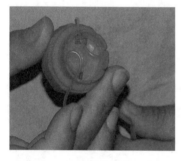
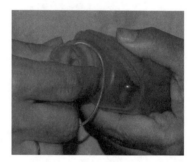

- Choose the desired tubing (slow flow – red valve, medium flow – white valve, fast flow – colorless valve).

- Hold the valve cover with the center projection upward, and place the valve over the center projection, matching the square projections on the valve with the cutouts on the cover (figure 84).

- Using the sides of the thumbs, carefully (to avoid tearing it) massage the valve downward onto the cover to cause it to sit flat and completely flush, without any space at all (figure 85). If there is any space or moisture between the valve and the valve cover, the device is likely to leak (figure 86).

- Gather the tubes and put them through the cap, from the thread end toward the end with multiple slits. Handle the tubes gently (figures 87, 88).

- Make sure the tubes are fully extended and that the tubes are cleared from the area between the cap and the valve cover.

HELPFUL TIPS

IF THE BABY GAGS OR OBJECTS TO THE FEELING OF THE TUBE, MARY ROSE TULLY, IBCLC, RECOMMENDS TAPING THE TUBE DIAGONALLY ALONG THE TOP LIP, HALF WAY BETWEEN THE PHILTRUM AND THE CORNER OF THE MOUTH.

HELPFUL TIPS

MARTA GUÓTH-GUMBERGER RECOMMENDS PURCHASING A HOOK AT A HARDWARE STORE TO MAKE IT EASIER TO ATTACH AND DETACH THE NECKLACE FROM THE SNS. BEAUTIFUL ILLUSTRATED INSTRUCTIONS FOR ASSEMBLY, INFORMATION ABOUT NUANCED USE, AND MANY CASE STUDIES ARE INCLUDED IN HER BOOKLET FOR PARENTS ON THE USE OF THE SNS (GUÓTH-GUMBERGER M., 2006).

- Snap the valve cover into the cap from the inner (thread) side (figure 89).

- Crimp off each tube in one of the slots in the cap, preferably keeping each tube on its own side of the cap so they can be identified at breast (figure 90).

- Fill the container with the desired amount of supplement.

- Screw the cap onto the threaded neck of the bottle, again being careful the tubing remains free (figure 91).

- Pinch the rope necklace and push it through the plastic loop at the back end of the container, loop it through itself to secure (like making a "Chinese" jump rope).

- Pull the necklace clasp back by pressing the inner button upward to free the gears from the rope.

- Place the necklace around the neck and adjust the cap to the desired height (at nipple height for neutral flow, above the nipples for faster flow, and below the nipples for slower flow).

The tubes can be taped to each breast, slid under the pad of a self-adhesive bandage on the breast, or one tube can be taped to the breast and the other tube taped up the side of the bottle and uncrimped to vent it faster than the tiny valves allow (figure 83). Venting one tube increases flow from the SNS.

Cleaning

Remove the rope necklace. Empty any leftover supplement. Rachel Brusseau (1998, unpublished study) analyzed human milk refrigerated in feeding bottles after use, and found little to no bacterial growth over 48 hours of storage. This indicates that expressed human can be refrigerated and reused once after contact with infant saliva.

Fill the container with hot, soapy water. Replace cap. Shake well to clean the inside of the container, then squeeze the container to force soapy water through the tubing. Repeat with clear water until all soap residue is removed. Then take apart the cap assembly and carefully clean the valve membrane, valve cover, and cap with soapy water and rinse well. Allow to air dry thoroughly before reassembly.

The manufacturer recommends boiling the device (container, tubes and valve assembly, valve cover and cap) once per day. Reduce the risk of melting the tubing by using a heavy saucepan and lining the bottom with a washcloth. Keep the tubing from contacting the walls or bottom of the pot.

Weaning

The amount of supplement offered per feeding can be gradually reduced. The infant can be encouraged to take less supplement by slowing the flow, either by using thinner tubing or lowering the device so the bottom of the cap is lower than the mother's nipples. This makes the infant work against gravity. When the amount of supplement per feeding is down to about ½ to 1 ounce, the SNS can be used at alternate feedings, and then discontinued if the infant continues to grow well and be content. More frequent breastfeeding can be expected as supplements are reduced, which helps to increase milk production.

Use

Assemble and fill the SNS as illustrated, and hang around the mother's neck. Lower the bottle until the cap is at nipple height. Uncrimp one tube, tape or hold to the breast, and latch the baby on. Adjust height and open or close the other tube as needed until optimal suck:swallow ratio is achieved (1:1; 2:1 for older infants). Allow the infant to take half the supplement at one breast, and if desired, change to the other breast for the second half. For infants who do well early in the feeding, but transfer less milk as they tire, the tube can be uncrimped once the infant stops swallowing.

Price

$29 wholesale, $56 retail

Contact Information

Medela, Inc. http://www.medelabreastfeedingus.com/
1.800.435.8316

Advantage

- Packed sterile
- Has two tubes, so can be taped in place for paired breastfeedings
- Durable (if treated with normal care)

- Reusable
- Effective

Disadvantages

- Assembly requires touching areas that will be in contact with milk
- Tubing unit tends to be delicate, particularly where the tubing enters the valve (spare tubing units are available by mail order).
- Most difficult supplementer device to assemble, but with practice it becomes easier.
- More dependent on gravity (but this can be used as a feature, see above)
- Requires a fairly competent baby, capable of generating some negative pressure during sucking

Suggested Uses

- Long term supplementation, especially when mother prefers this device or cannot afford replacement bags for the Lact-Aid.
- May allow breastfeeding for infants with inability to create full intraoral vacuum pressures, like those with poor soft palate seal with the posterior tongue
- Non-standard uses: Simultaneous feeding/supplementing of twins is shown in figure 92 – there are two tubes, two breasts, and two babies. It is very unlikely the infants are going to suck in synchrony, so they don't seem to interfere with each other's access to supplement.

Figure 92. Twins can be supplemented simultaneously with one SNS.

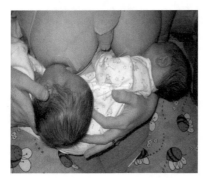

HELPFUL TIPS

MARTA GUÓTH-GUMBERGER, DIPL ING, IBCLC, WORKED WITH THE HAMICH FAMILY AND THEIR CLEFT-AFFECTED INFANT. BARBARA AND SVEN HAMICH WERE ABLE TO USE MARTA'S INFORMATION TO MODIFY THE SNS TO ALLOW AT BREAST FEEDING FOR THEIR INFANT (GUÓTH-GUMBERGER M., 2008). THEY MADE A HOLE IN THE CENTER OF THE LETTER "A" MOLDED INTO THE DEVICE. THE BABY WAS FED EXPRESSED MILK IN THE SUPPLEMENTER AND GIVEN ADDITIONAL SUPPORT TO MAINTAIN LATCH. BOTH TUBES WERE TAPED TO THE NIPPLE TO INCREASE FLOW, AS THE INFANT WAS UNABLE TO PRODUCE NEGATIVE PRESSURE. BARBARA COVERED THE HOLE WITH A FINGER TO STOP MILK FROM FLOWING, AND RELEASED THE FINGER BRIEFLY WHEN HER INFANT SUCKED. SHE EXPRESSED MILK REGULARLY TO PROVIDE MILK FOR THE MODIFIED SUPPLEMENTER. THE HAMICH'S ARE PLEASED TO SHARE THEIR TECHNIQUE TO HELP OTHER FAMILIES' BREASTFEED THEIR INFANTS WITH CLEFT PALATE, ILLUSTRATED IN FIGURES 93 AND 94.

Modification for Cleft-affected Infants

Figure 93. The Hamish's modification of the SNS for a cleft affected infant involves making a hole in the center of the molded "a" with a needle.

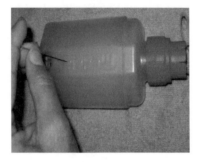

Figure 94. Barbara Hamish feeding her son.

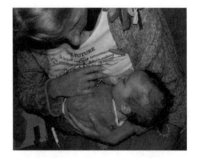

HELPFUL TIPS

CHRISTA HERZOG-ISLER, IBCLC, WORKED WITH AN INFANT WITH UNILATERAL CLEFT LIP AND PALATE (HERZOG-ISLER, 2008). SHE COLLABORATED WITH MARTA GUÓTH-GUMBERGER IN TEACHING THE HAMICH'S SNS MODIFICATION. THE INFANT'S MOTHER EXPRESSED MILK TO USE IN THE SNS AND WITH A HABERMAN FEEDER TO ENSURE GOOD GROWTH. A PALATAL OBTURATOR WAS TRIED, BUT DID NOT APPRECIABLY IMPROVE BREASTFEEDING. THOUGH THE BABY DID NOT TRANSFER MILK FROM THE BREAST, FEEDING MOST OF THE TIME AT BREAST ALLOWED HIM TO RETAIN A BREAST FOCUS. WITHIN TWO WEEKS OF HIS PALATE REPAIR AT FIVE MONTHS, HE WAS BREASTFEEDING EXCLUSIVELY.

Scales To Measure Milk Intake

Scales that are designed for test-weighing are precise to a few grams, and generally have the capacity to remember the initial weight and to calculate the change on re-weighing. If the baby is weighed immediately before and after the feeding in the same clothing, a good approximation of milk intake is displayed. Very young infants may be more comfortable if weighed prone or while swaddled in a blanket that has already been tared (weight subtracted from the scale).

Potential errors in the use of a scale include:

- Waiting too long after weighing to begin feeding (babies constantly lose weight by breathing out water vapor, over a short period of time this insensible water loss can be ignored).

- Changing the diaper before re-weighing if the baby urinates or stools (the urine or stool should weigh the same inside the baby or inside the diaper, as long as the diaper does not leak).

- Failing to account for socks or other small items of clothing that fall off the baby during feeding. Anything the baby was weighed with must go back on the scale with him.

- Failing to account for milk loss onto clothes. If baby dribbles milk during feeding, it's best to feed him only in a diaper, as milk soaking into his shirt will inflate the estimate of milk transferred.

- Failing to account for dripping onto the baby's clothing from the contra-lateral breast during MER (a tissue, nursing pad or small washcloth can be placed under mom's other nipple if it is exposed during the feeding and leaking is significant.

- Allowing a blanket or the baby's limbs to drape over the edge of the scale tray as in figure 95 – weights will be more accurate if the baby and any clothing or blankets are carefully gathered as close to the center of the scale tray as possible, like in figure 96.

Figure 95. Older infants can be difficult to weigh, an arm out of the scale basket can make test weighing inaccurate.

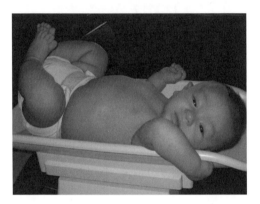

Figure 96. The blanket and infant are carefully contained within the scale basket on this BLB-12.

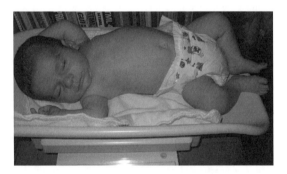

The amount of milk transferred at any one feeding by a thriving infant is irrelevant. Signs that an infant is drinking actively (wide eyed, intent expression, and long drawing one per second rhythmic sucking with a distinct pause as the jaw drops to create negative pressure in the mouth) are fairly reliable when working with healthy infants. However, when a child is not growing well, the information from a "snapshot" feeding can be clinically useful for determining whether interventions are effective and how much supplementation is needed. Babies with feeding problems may make gulping sounds (hard swallows), but transfer very little milk. Some babies are stealth swallowers, and it's difficult to hear them swallow without a stethoscope to the underside of their chin (cervical auscultation) as in figure 97. It is important to ask the mother if the feeding was typical, and if not, what was different. Perhaps the baby was not hungry or was overly challenged by the consultation. Small environmental changes can cause infants with sensory processing issues or prematurity to withdraw and may fail to elicit their best performance. To avoid disorganizing the baby during weighing, handle the baby gently, keep the baby's neck and shoulders contained and aligned during movement. Weighing the baby prone (laying on the belly) may be less stressful for the baby.

Figure 97. **Cervical auscultation or listening under the baby's chin for swallowing sounds**

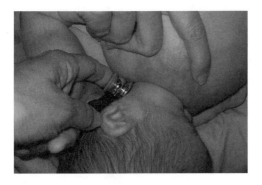

Scales for Test-Weighing
Tanita® BLB-12 (figures 98-99)

Figure 98. Tanita® BLB-12 scale, photo courtesy of Beth Shulman.

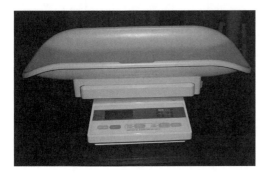

Figure 99. Tanita® BLB-12 control panel, photo courtesy of Beth Shulman.

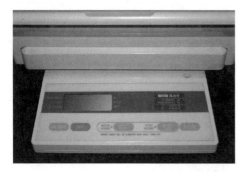

This scale has been discontinued and is no longer being supported. Replacement parts are not available, according to the director at Tanita's USA repair facility. While the scale is durable, no mechanical device lasts forever. LCs considering buying a used BLB-12 should consider the lack of replacement parts and repair. The BLB-12 was sold with an a/c adaptor included, it is a different adaptor than that used by the Medela BabyWeigh™, which is also manufactured by Tanita.

Technical specifications: precise to 2 grams under 12 pounds, and 5 grams between 12-24 pounds. Maximum capacity is 24 pounds. It can be set to weigh in either metric (grams) or Imperial (pounds and ounces) measurements. An optional carrying bag is available. The weight with 6 C cell batteries is around 13 pounds. This scale has a built in level, leveling legs, and is designed to compensate for infant movement.

Use

Place a clean blanket or cloth completely inside the scale basket, and press the on/tare button to start the scale disregarding the weight of the cloth. Place a clean diaper on the scale and press the on/tare button again to subtract the weight of the diaper, and dress the infant in this diaper. Place the baby on the scale. The scale will beep when the weight measurement stabilizes. Press the weight entry button, a mark will appear in the window next to memory weight. Remove the baby from the scale and feed. Immediately return the baby to the scale without changing the diaper. When the scale beeps, press the weight gain button. The weight gain will be displayed, and represents the amount of milk the infant consumed.

Price

Was around $600, has been discontinued.

Contact Information

http://www.tanita.com/en/

847.640.9241

Advantages

- First scale designed for test weighing
- Less expensive than the BabyWeigh.

Disadvantages

- No longer supported by repair and parts services.

Suggested Uses

- Test weighing of infants who are not growing well. Owners of the Tanita® BLB-12 can continue to use it as long as it continues to function. It will be difficult to repair as parts are no longer being manufactured.

Medela BabyWeigh™ Scale (formerly called Milky Weigh)

Figure 100. Medela BabyWeigh™ control panel, photo courtesy of Carol Chamblin.

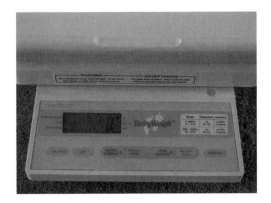

Medela product specialists offered assurances that this scale will continue to be sold and supported for the foreseeable future, and that if it is replaced, it will be replaced with a similar or better model. It is precise to 2 grams under 12 pounds, and 5 grams between 12- 24 pounds. It weighs about 13 pounds with the required 6 C batteries, or uses a proprietary a/c adaptor that is not included with the scale. The bag is available separately ($103.45). The scale requires calibration to maintain accuracy, calibration weight is sold separately ($65.59). It is designed to compensate for infant movement. It has a reweigh button, so the infant can be weighed again without being removed from the scale, and can change between Imperial and metric measures as well.

Use

Place a clean cloth, blanket or paper towel on the scale if desired. Turn scale on. This will zero the weight of the cloth the baby will lay on. If desired, place a clean diaper on the scale and press the on/zero button to tare the weight of the diaper. Dress the baby in only this diaper for a "naked weight" without the risk of mess. Place the baby on the scale and wait for the scale to beep to indicate the weight reading has stabilized. Press the weight entry button to save the pre-feeding weight. Immediately after feeding and in the same diaper, weigh the baby again. Press the weight gain button. The change in weight will be displayed, and represents the baby's milk intake. If the baby's movement makes the weight unreliable, press the reweigh button without removing the baby from the scale.

Price

$989.49 - scale, $103.45 – bag, $65.59 – calibration weight

Contact Information

Medela, Inc.   http://www.medelabreastfeedingus.com/

1.800.435.8316

Advantages

- Designed for test weighing

Disadvantages

- More expensive than other scales manufactured by Tanita

Suggested Uses

- Weighing infants who are not growing well to determine milk intake in comparison to the amount of milk the mother can express.

Tanita® BD-815U

Figure 101. Tanita® BD-815U

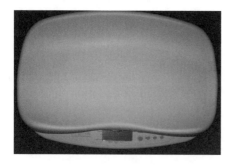

Figure 102. Tanita® BD-815U control panel

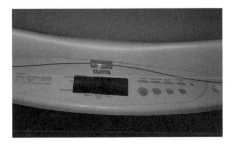

The Tanita® BD-815U is designed for preterm infants and infants with growth and feeding difficulties. It is lighter than BLB-12/BabyWeigh, weighs around 10 pounds, uses fewer and smaller batteries (4 AA cells), communicates with a computer so automated charting and graphing are possible, has higher max weight capacity (33 pounds versus 24 pounds), and better memory function. Larger, more stable base, lower profile tray reduces risk of baby falling, but requires more space. Extend mode allows weighing in one gram increments for the entire weight range of the scale. Does not require calibration, comes with a three year warranty. Case (model 110) is almost 4 pounds, but has pockets for files and scale liners. The fit in the carrying bag is very tight; the scale fits best with the front (the controls) at the back of the bag. The BD-815U comes with a soft, replaceable, washable cover to protect the scale surface and cushion the baby. It has memory and recall functions, as well as automatic weight gain calculation. The auto-stabilization feature helps improve accuracy when infants move during weighing. It has leveling legs and a built in level indicator (scales are most reliable when level). The a/c adaptor is included in the purchase price.

Use

Place a clean cloth, towel or blanket on the scale. Toddler size cloth diapers are particularly useful for this purpose and can be sanitized by washing in hot water. Press the on/tare button. When the scale displays 0, place a clean diaper on the scale, and press on/tare again to subtract the weight of the diaper. Dress the baby in the diaper, and place the baby on the scale. When the scale beeps, press the grey memory button. Feed the infant, and return to the scale. When the scale beeps, press the grey weight gain button. The weight displayed when the scale beeps indicates the weight of the milk the baby consumed. If more precision is required during weighing, press the extend button to weigh to 1 gram. This scale also has advanced memory functions, and interfaces with a computer to perform data capture and graphing. See the illustrated manufacturer's instruction book for use of the advanced features.

Price

$840 – scale, $66.40 – carrying bag

Contact Information

http://www.tanita.com/en/

847.640.9241

Advantages

- Designed for test weighing of infants requiring intensive care
- Flat tray improves infant's stability during weighing
- Larger capacity and maximum weight allows test weighing of toddlers
- Easier to carry and handle, has handles at the sides of the base.
- Stable, base is the same size as the basket
- Three year warranty

Disadvantages

- Takes slightly more room than the BLB-12/BabyWeigh

Suggested Uses

- Best for accurate test weights of vulnerable infants, including preterm babies and those with feeding difficulties.

Breast Pumps

The same characteristics that make infant sucking effective apply to breast pump effectiveness: production of appropriate negative pressures, prevention of nipple compression or distortion, and smooth cycling between pressures. Smoother coordination between the individual movements of sucking is responsible for the increased efficiency of babies at breastfeeding as they mature (Lau & Schanler, 1996). The combination of smooth cycling and appropriate negative pressure seems to differentiate effective breast pumps from less effective ones.

Normal infants have significant flexibility in their sucking behavior and will experiment until they find a pattern that works best for their individual mother. Unfortunately, breast pumps do not have as much flexibility. While some mothers can effectively "empty" their breasts with any pump, some require more negative pressure or a different cycle speed. Lactation consultants are often called on to help when a client's pump is not meeting her needs. Sometimes the assembly or use of the pump can be corrected or refined, and sometimes the mother needs a different pump. As of this writing, the FDA has not developed standards for breast pump effectiveness. There is a growing body of research and clinical experience that can be used to provide information to help guide choices for mothers having difficulty.

The first consideration is the reason the mother is using the pump. If she needs to collect milk for occasional brief separation from her baby, the choice of pump is less critical than if she is pumping all the milk her preterm or ill baby requires. The amount of time required at each pumping session is another factor to consider. Hand pumps and electric pumps with smaller motors may require 50-100% more time to 'empty' the breast than a hospital grade pump does. This time constraint becomes a greater concern when mothers need to use the pump many times a day and when they have other demands on their time. The percentage of available milk the pump can remove is another important consideration. The more dependent the mother is on the pump for milk removal, the more critical it is that the pump removes at least as much milk as a healthy breastfeeding infant in 10-20 minutes when used with a dual kit.

Nipple comfort and safety is important for all mothers. The pump flange must fit snugly against the breast and the nipple tunnel must be wide enough to allow the nipple to expand when negative pressure is applied to it. If the sides of the nipple rub against the tunnel edges, there can be friction injury. The pump must allow free movement of the nipple at the junction of the areola to avoid injury. If the nipple is barely moving and the mother has pain, the flange likely touches her breast at the junction of the nipple and areola. The flange must also allow the nipple to perfuse properly. Discoloration of the breast during pumping, such as purple nipples or a white or red line at the base of the nipple, indicates that the nipple tunnel is impeding blood flow. Figure 103 illustrates darkening of the nipple and a white ring at the base of the nipple in a mother pumping with a flange that is too small. Fortunately, pump manufacturers now make a variety of flanges/breast shields for improved fit.

Figure 103. Even this larger flange is too small for this mother, note the white ring at the base of the nipple and the dusky nipple from impeded blood flow.

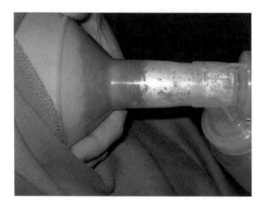

It is important to understand that the maximum vacuum of a breast pump will be reduced if the flange has a larger airspace than the standard flange. Each breast pump motor is calibrated to work with the amount of airspace in the expected collection kit, so using a different flange or kit may change the pressure at the nipple to either too low to be effective or too high to be safe for skin integrity. If using non-standard equipment, it is wise to test with a vacuum gauge and instruct mothers to turn down the vacuum if the pump is uncomfortable. One reason that some mothers may be more comfortable with larger flanges or with inserts like Pumpin Pals (page 158) is that these items lower the vacuum on the nipple. It is important to ensure that the lowered vacuum is still effective.

Choosing a Breast Pump

The choice of pump is less important when it will only be used casually and infrequently because any milk left in the breast by the pump can be consumed by the baby at the next feeding and potential reduction of milk production is low. When a pump is used frequently or exclusively, it is vital that the pump empties the breast reliably and efficiently. Babies communicate hunger and cry if their subtler communications go unanswered, but mothers need to be vigilant to pump often enough to build and maintain an adequate milk supply. A healthy baby whose mother's milk production lags behind his needs will feed more frequently and perhaps for longer to empty the breast better. Pump-dependant mothers need to keep track of their milk production and use similar strategies if milk production is less than needed.

Norms for Milk Production

It is important to use the full term infant as the norm and not just pump for the current needs of a preterm infant because milk production is calibrated in the early days or weeks after birth. Research-based milk output goals when pumping for a preterm infant are about 500 ml per day by the second week (3500 g per week), as all mothers expressing this much milk by week 2 had sufficient milk at 4 and 5 weeks as well (Hill et al., 1999). Simultaneous pumping and a very brief breast massage before simultaneous pumping (Jones et al., 2001), along with an early start to expression (within 6 hours of birth) were important. Moreover, day 4 pumped volume greater than 395 ml for the day improved the prognosis for sufficient milk production at week 6 for mothers of preterm infants (Hill & Aldag, 2005). In Hill and Aldag's (2005) sample, mothers were instructed to use the pump (Lactina Select) simultaneously for at least 10 minutes, for 2 minutes past the last drops, at least 8 times a day, and after stimulating their MER. Three out of 27 mothers who produced less than 140 ml on day 4 were able to make sufficient milk by 6 weeks with consistent pumping 6-8 times daily and a lack of expressed stress. Likewise, 3 of the 27 mothers pumping more than 395 ml on day 4 postpartum did not make sufficient milk by 6 weeks, all experienced major stressors (Hill & Aldag, 2005).

In my own practice, I encourage pump-dependent mothers to initially aim for significantly more milk than we expect their infant to need. This excess capacity makes milk production less vulnerable to occasional stresses or missed expression sessions, and has helped mothers of infants with cleft palate and genetic disorders provide their milk for their infants for up to 2 years.

How Breast Pumps Work

Just as negative pressure in the infant's mouth moves milk from the breast with the assistance of increased positive pressure from the milk ejection reflex and the force exerted by milk in the ducts, negative pressure in the nipple tunnel of the pump provides the impetus for milk removal. Several manufacturers experimented with using compression on the breast along with negative pressure in their pumps, but these were not commercially successful.

HELPFUL TIPS

POWER PUMPING

POWER PUMPING IS A STRATEGY DEVELOPED BY KATE SHARP, IBCLC, AND I, AND NAMED BY LEIGH ANNE O'CONNOR, IBCLC. IT MIMICS THE "CLUSTER FEEDING" THAT INFANTS DO TO INCREASE MATERNAL MILK PRODUCTION. MOMS ARE ENCOURAGED TO PLACE THEIR PUMP IN THE ROOM THEY SPEND THE MOST TIME IN AND TO USE IT EVERY TIME THEY PASS IT OR HAVE A MOMENT TO SIT. IF THE BABY IS HEALTHY AND FULL TERM, THEY ARE ENCOURAGED TO PUT A CLEAN TOWEL OR DIAPER OVER THE KIT BETWEEN USES AND CLEAN THE KIT ABOUT EVERY 4 HOURS, AS HUMAN MILK IS SAFE AT ROOM TEMPERATURE FOR AT LEAST THAT LONG. THEY ARE INSTRUCTED TO GET A NAP DURING THE DAY IF AT ALL POSSIBLE, AND TO POWER PUMP FOR ONLY A FEW DAYS AT A TIME. A SPOUSE'S DAYS OFF OR DAYS WHEN THERE IS OTHER HELP AVAILABLE ARE IDEAL FOR POWER PUMPING. USUALLY 2-3 DAYS OF VERY FREQUENT PUMPING (ABOUT EVERY 45-120 MINUTES DURING THE DAY AND AT LEAST ONCE AT NIGHT) YIELDS A SUBSTANTIAL INCREASE IN MILK PRODUCTION, AND MOM CAN RESUME HER PREVIOUS PUMPING ROUTINE OR STEP BACK TO 7-8 EXPRESSIONS PER DAY.

I will focus on hospital grade pumps because they are most pertinent to solving breastfeeding problems in lactation consultant practice. For a broader look at breast pumps, I recommend Marsha Walker's excellent overview and critique of the research (Walker, 2005).

Safety and Effectiveness

Modern breast pumps limit vacuum to prevent the potential for nipple damage. Suction parameters for pump safety were developed in 1939 when the Abt pump reportedly caused nipple skin rupture in 33% of users (Egnell, 1956). Both peak negative pressure and the amount of time the nipple was subjected to negative pressure were important in producing nipple damage. Einar Egnell, a civil engineer in Sweden, designed the Sister Maya's Breast Pump (now known as the Ameda SMB) to expose nipple skin to far less than the one second of consecutive negative pressure and lower overall pressures than the Abt pump produced to eliminate the risk of skin damage. The original SMB's peak negative pressure was -200 mmHg.

Egnell clearly understood that filling of the breast stopped milk production at an internal pressure of 28 mmHg, which balances the pressure that the musculature around the nipple exerts to keep milk in. The milk ejection reflex then increases the pressure inside the breast, while the infant (or pump) exerts negative pressure to overcome the resistance of the nipple to milk release. The lower pressure outside the nipple and higher pressure inside causes milk to flow toward the lower pressure.

Egnell also cleverly measured hourly output in a mother pumping for her preterm infant and found that 40% of milk was made in the first hour, 35% in the second hour, 20% in the third, and only 5% in the fourth. This phenomenon of reduced milk production speed as the breast fills was not well appreciated in English-speaking countries until recently, and explains why expressing every one to two hours maximizes milk yield over expressing every three hours or less frequently.

Recent research shows that the most milk is removed by a breast pump when the mother used the highest suction pressure that was comfortable (Kent et al., 2008). Unfortunately, a substantial proportion of successfully breastfeeding mothers in the study failed to remove 50-70% of the milk in their breasts as calculated by comparing fore and hind milk fat content. The authors postulate that duct width or other breast characteristics may be responsible for this finding, but it is equally likely that these mothers require more than the -270mmHg peak suction of the study pump, a different suction curve, or a different way to stimulate their milk ejection reflex. The type of massage found to increase milk yield in pumping mothers by Jones' group consisted of gently rolling the knuckles down the breast from ribcage to areola and nipple (Jones et al., 2001). This massage was chosen because it gave tactile stimulation without manually expressing milk, which would have interfered with the study results.

Indeed, manual expression can be more effective than electric breast pump use in the expression of colostrum during the first 48 hours. A crossover study of 15 mothers expressed by experienced hospital staff either manually or with a Symphony pump every 3 hours starting 6 hours after birth found manual expression removed twice the milk (Ohyama et al., 2007) over 7 trials of each method for each woman. The downside of manual expression by a health care professional was that significantly more women found it painful versus pumping. It is unknown if manual expression is more effective than every hospital grade breast pump before lactogenesis II, but many lactation consultants recommend manual expression followed by electric breast pump use in the first 2 days after birth.

Jane Morton, MD, IBCLC, found that adding manual expression to electric breast pumping (a technique she calls Hands-On Pumping) likewise increases milk production by facilitating breast emptying (http://newborns.stanford.edu/Breastfeeding/MaxProduction.html). She recommends that mothers double pump until milk stops flowing, and then switch to either single pumping with breast massage or manual expression to fully empty the breasts. In the colostral phase, Dr. Morton recommends frequent hand expression to moms of preterm infants until lactogenesis II, and then switching to the hands-on pumping strategy previously explained. The use of a small container, such as a Snappies sterile colostrum collector (figure 104) or a small medicine cup, helps normalize typical volumes of colostrum for mothers. Figure 105 shows a mother manually expressing colostrum into a sterile test tube which is stocked by the hospital for multiple purposes.

Figure 104. Snappies makes two sizes of inexpensive, sterile colostrum collection containers, a 13 ml one for use with manual expression (foreground) and a 30 ml one for use with an electric breast pump (background).

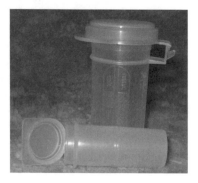

Figure 105. Manual expression of colostrum into an appropriate sized container. Photo courtesy of Esther D. Grunis.

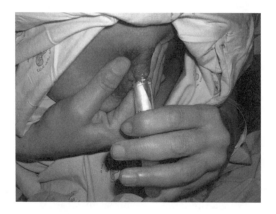

If an electric pump is used during the early days after birth, substituting a smaller container between the valve and the bottle or instead of the bottle may reduce loss of colostrum in the tubing, and reduce maternal dissatisfaction with the amount pumped. Ameda diaphragms used this way can then be used as feeding cups, or milk can be drawn up in a syringe because it does not stick to the silicone material. This technique can be used in either company's kit. Figures 106 through 109 illustrate this innovation by a mother of a preterm infant. Now several companies make small sterile containers for collecting colostrum. These are covered in the section on pumping accessories (page 153).

Figure 106. A spare silicone diaphragm is inserted into the top of the collection bottle.

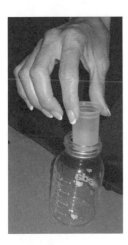

Figure 107. The rim holds it in place.

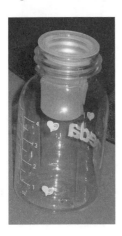

Figure 108. The collection kit is screwed on. The thin silicone does not disrupt the seal in the kit.

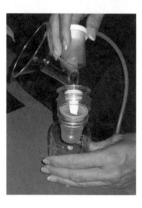

Figure 109. Ready for use

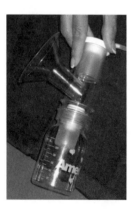

Clinicians have found that use of older, metal piston pumps sometimes increases pumped milk yield markedly for mothers struggling to pump with newer pumps. Dee Kassing, IBCLC, thought of a way to test this hypothesis without disrupting the mother by switching the pump end of the collection kit tubing between a Symphony and a Classic pump as the mother expressed.

The take-home message here is that mothers differ in their vacuum needs during pumping, and so far no one pump has been developed that works optimally for absolutely all mothers. If a pumping mother is having difficulty with her milk production despite sufficient pumping frequency, the clinician should first check the kit to ensure that it is assembled correctly and that no parts are worn; then check the pump to ensure that it is operating correctly and producing the expected vacuum pressures; and finally check the mother's technique and the fit of the flanges. If major improvements cannot be made, try switching to a pump with a higher vacuum

HELPFUL TIPS

DEE'S PUMP TRIAL METHOD

THE SAME PUMP DOESN'T WORK BEST FOR EVERY MOTHER. FOR THOSE USING A HOSPITAL-GRADE RENTAL PUMP, A LOT OF MOTHERS DO FINE WITH THE MEDELA SYMPHONY. HOWEVER, I HAVE ALSO WORKED WITH NUMEROUS MOTHERS WHO GET A LOT MORE MILK USING THE OLDER MEDELA CLASSIC. (AMEDA RENTAL PUMPS AREN'T FOUND IN MY AREA.)

I USE THE FOLLOWING SYSTEM TO DETERMINE WHICH PUMP IS THE BETTER PUMP TO RENT TO A PARTICULAR MOTHER. FIRST, I CHECK THE FLANGE FIT TO BE SURE THE MOTHER IS USING THE PROPER SIZE. I USUALLY USE THE CLASSIC TO DETERMINE CORRECT FLANGE SIZE BECAUSE IT HOLDS ITS SUCTION LEVEL AT THE SAME POINT EVEN WHEN TURNED OFF TO CHANGE FLANGE SIZES, SO IS EASIER FOR MOTHERS TO COMPARE THE FEEL OF ONE SIZE FLANGE AGAINST ANOTHER AT THE SAME SUCTION LEVEL. THE SYMPHONY DOESN'T WORK THIS WAY. NOT ALL MOTHERS CAN USE A PUMP AT THE HIGHEST SUCTION LEVEL COMFORTABLY, SO ONCE THE MOTHER HAS THE CORRECT SIZE FLANGE AND THE CLASSIC IS SET AT THE MOTHER'S HIGHEST COMFORTABLE SUCTION LEVEL, I SET UP BOTH A CLASSIC AND A SYMPHONY WITHIN EASY REACH OF THE MOTHER. I SET THE SYMPHONY AT A SIMILAR LEVEL OF SUCTION (ESTIMATED, BASED ON NUMBER OF BARS IN SYMPHONY WINDOW VERSUS SUCTION LEVEL SETTING OF THE CLASSIC). I TURN ON BOTH PUMPS AND LET THE MOTHER AGAIN EXPERIENCE A FEW SUCKS WITH THE CLASSIC, SINCE THE MOTHER WAS USING THAT PUMP FOR THE FLANGE-SIZE TEST. THEN I SIMPLY MOVE THE TUBE FROM THE CLASSIC TO THE SYMPHONY AND ASK THE MOTHER WHICH FEELS BETTER. I HAVE THE MOTHER EXPERIENCE A FEW SUCKS WITH THE SYMPHONY, AND THEN I MOVE THE TUBE BACK AND FORTH BETWEEN THE PUMPS UNTIL THE MOTHER IS SURE WHICH ONE FEELS BETTER OR WE CAN TELL THAT ONE PUMP YIELDS NOTICEABLY MORE MILK.

SOME MOTHERS LIKE THE SUCK-FEEL OF ONE PUMP OVER THE OTHER. SOME CAN USE A HIGHER SUCTION LEVEL MORE COMFORTABLY ON ONE PUMP RATHER THAN THE OTHER. BUT SOMETIMES IT IS VERY EASY TO SEE THAT ONE PUMP PRODUCES A LOT MORE MILK IN A SIMILAR AMOUNT OF TIME. IT MAY BE THAT ONE PUMP YIELDS DROPS AND THE OTHER PUMP YIELDS SQUIRTS. IT MAY BE THAT ONE PUMP PULLS ONE MILK STREAM FROM THE NIPPLE PORES WHILE THE OTHER PUMP PULLS THREE OR FOUR MILK STREAMS AT THE SAME TIME. FOR MOTHERS WHO DON'T YET HAVE ENOUGH MILK TO YIELD SQUIRTS DURING PUMPING, I FIND THAT THE PUMP THE MOTHER CONSIDERS MOST COMFORTABLE USUALLY YIELDS THE BETTER MILK SUPPLY. AS WITH ANYTHING IN LIFE, THERE ARE EXCEPTIONS. SO FAR, I HAVE WORKED WITH TWO MOTHERS WHO LIKED THE FEEL OF THE SYMPHONY MUCH BETTER, BUT DESPITE SEVERAL DAYS OF PUMPING WITH THE SYMPHONY JUST COULDN'T GET ENOUGH MILK FOR THEIR BABIES UNTIL THEY SWITCHED TO THE CLASSIC. DEE KASSING, IBCLC pressure. Conversely, if a mother's nipples become damaged during pumping, check the pump with a vacuum gauge. The Medela Classic™ has a pressure regulator that sometimes goes out of adjustment, and pressures of -400 mmHg have been noted in rare instances. The pump can easily be adjusted back to the -280 mmHg range by a repair technician. Lower than normal (-140 mmHg) peak vacuums have also been observed. Ideally, all electric breast pumps should be checked with a pressure gauge between rental clients to ensure that the motor is functioning within expected parameters for the model.

Table 3: Ameda Breastfeeding Products (All values are for double pumping with standard flange size.)

Model	Minimum suction	Maximum suction	Kit used	Flange sizes available
SMB*	-100 mmHg or less	At least -230 mmHg (Up to -280 or -300)	All Ameda pumps use the same kit (Hygeinikit)	21 (soft silicone, Flexishield) 22.5 (reducing insert) 25 mm (standard) 28.5 (reducing insert) 30.5 32.5 (reducing insert) 36 mm
Lact-e*	-100 mmHg or less	At least -230 mmHg (Up to -280 or -300)		
Elite*	-60 mmHg or less On Maximum cycles	At least -200 mmHg On Maximum cycles		

Table 4. Medela Breastfeeding Products (All values are for double pumping with standard flange size.)

Model	Minimum suction	Maximum suction	Kit used	Flange sizes available
Classic™	-80 to -120	-220 to -280	Kit discontinued, barrier filter will still be sold and can covert other Medela kits to use with Classic pump	21 mm 24 mm (standard) 24 mm SoftFit 27 mm 30 mm
Lactina*	-90 to -120 (can vary 10 mmHg with increased speed)	-200 to -240 (can vary 10 mmHg with increased speed)	Lactina Double Pumping System or Symphony and Lactina Double Pumping system	36 mm 40 mm (glass breast shield, $70 each wholesale)
Symphony*	-40 at 1 bar -60 at 1 drop	-240 to -255 at 16 bars -210 at 16 drops (2 samples had peak suction less than -200)	Symphony and Lactina (combination) Double Pumping System	Modular connector required to change flanges (standard on permanent kits, not supplied in disposable hospital kits)

Knowledge of the suction parameters of the different breast pumps is also important for special maternal situations. Sore nipples have reduced skin integrity and injured skin is more vulnerable to pressure-induced injury. Nipple elasticity is reduced during engorgement because the swollen breast fills out the skin more, reducing the amount of slack available for normal nipple movement during feeding and pumping. Linda Pohl, PE, IBCLC, studied suction characteristics of breast pumps and recommended the lower minimum suction pressures of the Ameda Elite while pumping for engorgement and sore nipples. She recommends hospital grade pumps with large motors that produce a smooth suction curve and higher maximum suction pressure for pump dependant mothers, for whom the most complete breast emptying is essential (Pohl, 2003). Pohl also found that the suction curves differed for each pump, even within a brand. The Ameda SMB and Lact-e had smooth suction curves with a slight hold at the maximum vacuum; the Medela Classic had a smooth suction curve with a faster release (more like a sine wave). While the hospital grade breast pumps all work for most mothers, some individuals will get significantly more milk with one suction curve over another.

Another difference between pump brands is whether there is a neutral rest phase or a positive pressure rest phase. A neutral rest phase (used by Medela pumps) releases all pressure changes, allowing the nipple to be exposed to only environmental pressures. A positive pressure rest phase (used by Ameda pumps) uses a minimal positive pressure to push the nipple away from the nipple tunnel to facilitate refilling. Again, both patterns are effective for most mothers, but one may work better than the other for certain individuals.

Hospital Grade Pumps

Ameda Elite®

The Elite® (figures 110 and 111) is designed to allow continuously variable vacuum and cycle settings that are independent of each other, so each mother can find her own optimal setting. Vacuum is provided by a plastic piston, which is pulled open at a speed and depth controlled by an internal computer in response to the settings of the two dials. It is recommended that mothers start on the highest cycles and lowest vacuum until the MER occurs (a drop of milk will appear on the nipples), then turn the cycles down to somewhere in the medium range and turn the vacuum up as high as needed to get sprays of milk from both breasts. If the vacuum becomes uncomfortable, mom can either reduce the vacuum slightly or reduce the cycle speed slightly, since they are independently controllable. The piston is exposed, and if it becomes dirty, the smoothness of the suction curve will be affected. The piston can be easily changed by the rental station as illustrated in figures 112 through 116. Elite breast pumps are also available with a vermin-proof cover over the piston, which keeps the piston clean and prevents cockroach entry. The electric cord conveniently winds around the back of the pump in a designated area. The dials are made of plastic and sometimes strip. If they seem to spin easily, but this does not affect the settings, they are easily replaceable by the rental depot by just pulling the old ones off, lining up the new dials with the stem, and pressing them on. The holder in the dial is shaped to provide proper placement on the stem (figure 117).

Figure 110. Ameda Elite breast pump

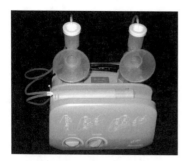

Figure 111. Elite's control panel

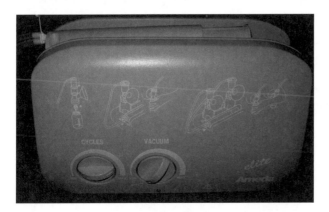

Figures 112-116: Changing the Elite piston

Figure 112. Elite with the piston removed, showing the stationary rod (left) and the moveable arm (right)

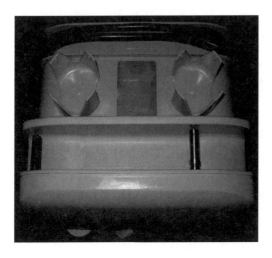

Figure 113. Place the end of the inner piston cylinder over the black stationary arm on the left.

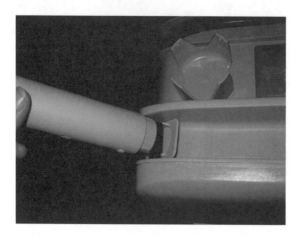

Figure 114. Rotate the piston into place and press down to seat well.

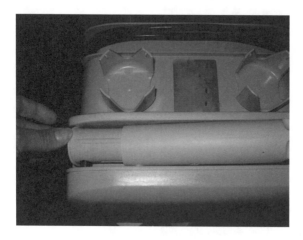

Figure 115. Extend the piston's outer cylinder until the notch in the underside reaches the silver moveable arm on the right.

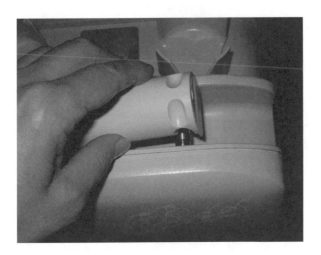

Figure 116. Press down firmly until the cylinder is well seated on the moveable arm.

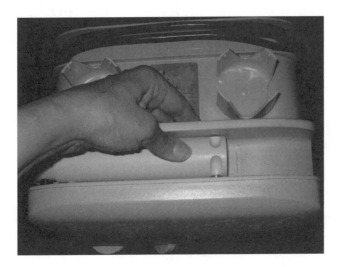

Figure 117. Elite dials

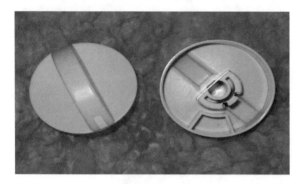

Price

Approximately $650-$750 wholesale, $1000 retail. (internal rechargeable battery $150 additional) Available to rental depots for $14-18 per month, depending on number of pumps rented ($5 additional for internal battery).

Contact

Ameda Breastfeeding Products http://www.ameda.com

1.866.99.AMEDA

Ameda Lact-e®

Figure 118. Ameda Lact-e breast pump

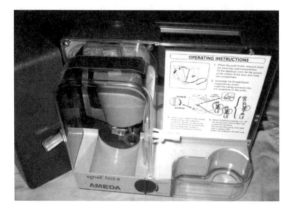

Figure 119. Lact-e with dual hygeinikit

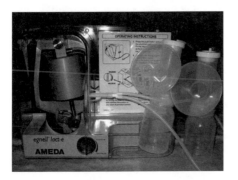

The Lact-e® has a metal motor and piston very similar to the Ameda SMB®, which is fitted into a portable case. The suction curve is smooth with a slight "hold" at the peak, and a positive pressure rest phase when the negative pressure is released. Lact-e's are still being repaired, but they are no longer being manufactured. Ameda hopes to replace them with the Platinum pump, with a similar suction curve in a lighter weight design.

Price

Discontinued, still available to rental depots at $16-$21 per month, depending on number rented.

Contact

Ameda Breastfeeding Products http://www.ameda.com

1.866.99.AMEDA

Ameda SMB®

Figure 120. Ameda SMB, photo courtesy of Rachel Myr.

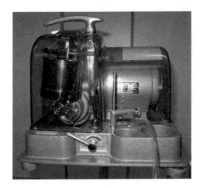

The SMB® is the original Egnell breast pump. Suction is derived from a rotating metal piston, creating a smooth suction curve with a slightly flattened peak and a positive pressure rest period after the suction is released. Most of the internal parts are metal, leading to a long lasting machine. Many SMB's are still in use in hospitals around the world. This pump is being phased out as parts are becoming difficult to obtain.

Ameda Kit Assembly

Ameda pumps use the same kit. Figures 121 through 129 illustrate the assembly and alteration for single and double pumping of the Ameda hygeinikit.

Price

Discontinued, still available to rental depots at $16-$22 per month, depending on number of pumps rented.

Contact

Ameda Breastfeeding Products http://www.ameda.com

1.866.99.AMEDA

Figure 121. The pump body or flange (left) and the duckbill style one piece valve (right)

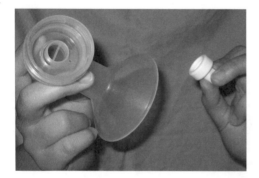

Figure 122. Handling the valve by the thicker sides, fit it onto the circular projection on the underside of the pump body.

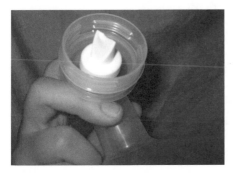

Figure 123. The silicone diaphragm is placed solid side down in the top of the pump body.

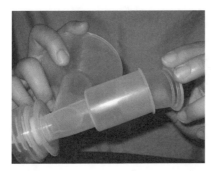

Figure 124. The diaphragm in place

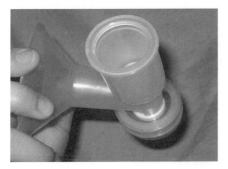

Figure 125. The adapter cap is pressed down until an audible click is heard.

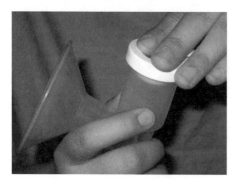

Figure 126. A collection container is screwed onto the threads.

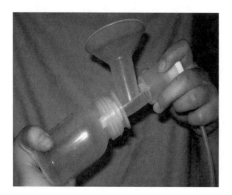

Figure 127. For double pumping, both tubes should be connected to the tubing adapter.

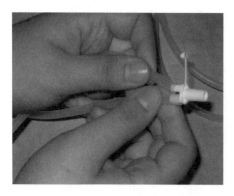

Figure 128. For single pumping, the upper tube can be removed and the pin closed; but suction will not be reduced if both sides are assembled and only one side is used.

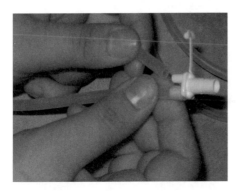

Figure 129. Make sure to close the pin in the adapter if one tube has been removed.

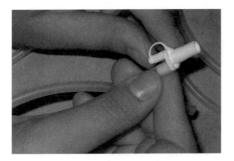

Medela Classic™

KATHY MIRRA, IBCLC, RECOMMENDS CAREFUL EXAMINATION OF THE BARRIER/FILTER IF A MOTHER IS HAVING POOR RESULTS WITH A CLASSIC PUMP. NEW BARRIER FILTERS WILL APPEAR MILKY WHITE, WITH A CONSISTENT COLOR THROUGHOUT. FILTERS THAT HAVE GOTTEN WET OR BEEN TOUCHED WILL HAVE A THINNER OR UNEVEN WHITE COATING, OR EVEN A GRAYISH TINGE. FIGURE 132 SHOWS A SUBOPTIMAL BARRIER FILTER ON THE LEFT AND A NEW, FUNCTIONAL ONE ON THE RIGHT.

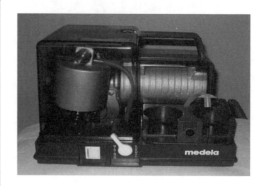

Figure 130. Medela Classic™ breast pump, photo courtesy of Kathleen Mirra.

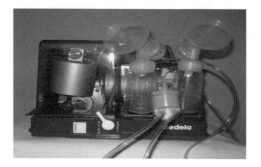

Figure 131. Classic™ with dual kit, photo courtesy of Kathleen Mirra.

The Classic™ pump has a metal piston and a smooth suction curve with a very short peak – like a sine wave in shape. It is being discontinued because parts are no longer available for repairs. Rental prices to depots have risen to $39 per month, and Classic and universal kits are no longer being manufactured. The Classic barrier/filter is still available for rental stations to use in adapting Lactina kits to the Classic. Adapting a Symphony kit requires the purchase of a pump connector, as well as the barrier/filter. Rental stations using the separately purchased barrier filters may wish to check the suction before issuing them to mothers, as lactation consultants in various parts of the U.S. have recently received defective barrier filters that reduced pumping pressures below effective ranges.

Figure 132. Worn barrier filter (left) and effective one (right). Photo courtesy of Kathy Mirra.

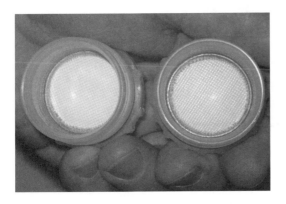

Classic™ kit assembly

Figures 133-135. Classic™ connector and barrier/filter. Photos courtesy of Kathy Mirra.

Figure 133.

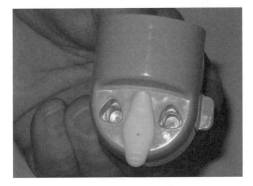

Figure 134.

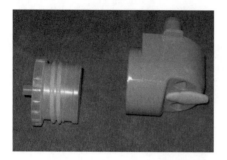

Figure 135.

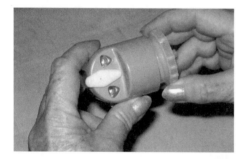

The same pump connector (figures 133 and 134) is used for both the Lactina® and the Classic™ breast pumps, but it is used in different ways. When using the connector with the Classic, the colorless barrier/filter is screwed into the threads of the yellow connector (figure 135), and the circular projection on the yellow connector is pressed into the hole in the pump. The pump's main tube is then attached to the small tube at the solid end of the barrier/filter as shown in figure 131, and the collection kit tubing is attached to the two holes in the connector. If the pump is only going to be used singly, the port plug is removed from the holder (center hole) and rotated to cover the unused hole.

When the connector is used for the Lactina® pump, the flat tab on the right side of the yellow connector (figure 133) is slid into the slot on the left front of the pump. This is vital to stabilizing the piston for proper operation.

Price

Discontinued. Rental depots who already have them are being charged $39 per month, payable annually.

Contact

Medela, Inc. http://www.medelabreastfeedingus.com/

1.800.435.8316

Medela Lactina®

Figure 136. Lactina® Breast Pump with kit, photo courtesy of Denise Altman.

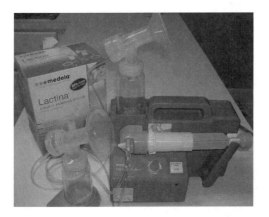

The Lactina® (figure 136) uses an exterior piston to provide suction. There are three suction settings - minimum, medium, and maximum; and in the later models (Select), there are several speed settings as well. The Lactina was designed to be a lighter weight, lower cost alternative for mothers who need to pump frequently. There are fewer settings and the suction curve is less smooth than other hospital grade pumps, so if a pump-dependant mother has difficulty with milk production using the Lactina, she might do better with a different pump. Many employed mothers whose infants' breastfeed at home find the Lactina effective.

Lactina® Assembly

Figures 137-142.   Assembling the Lactina kit, photos courtesy of Denise Altman.

Figure 137.

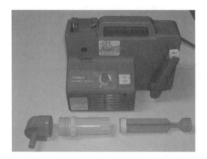

Figure 138.

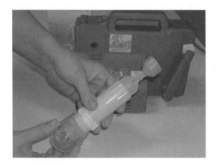

Figure 139.

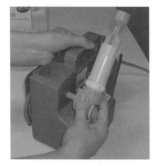

Figure 140.

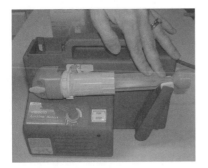

Figure 141.

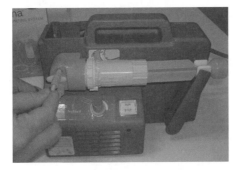

Figure 142.

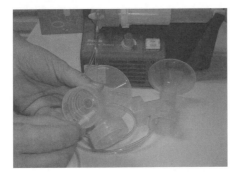

- Assembling the piston (figure 137) – Ensure that the rubber piston seal is on the base of the inner piston, with the wider end pointing to the narrowed handle of the piston. Place the handle end of the inner piston through the threaded end of the outer one and push through the corrugated end.

- Screw the assembled piston into the pump connector (figure 138). The Lactina® pump connector is identical to the one for the Classic™.

- Push the cylinder at the back of the pump connector into the hole at the left front of the pump (figure 139), then rotate the piston to the right to catch the flat projection on the connector (figure 133) in the slot on the pump. This is important for stabilizing the piston.

- Extend the inner piston and press the narrowed area into the rubber holder on the moveable arm of the pump (figure 140).

- Press the yellow triangular ends of the kit tubing into the ports on the pump connector as shown in figure 141. Note that the port plug is in the center (holder) position. If single pumping, move the port plug to cover the unused port and press it in firmly.

- Insert the narrower, circular cross section ends of the kit tubing into the holes in the back of the pump connector (figure 142). These are usually transparent, but are beige on some kits.

- Continue assembling the breast flange/shield, valve and valve membrane, and collection container onto the pump connector as illustrated in figures 147-151.

- Set the speed dial to a medium to high speed, and spin the vacuum regular ring to select the desired vacuum. I recommend starting on high speed and low vacuum until the milk ejection reflex is stimulated, and then slowing the speed to medium and raising the vacuum as needed until milk sprays from both breasts.

Price

Rents for $14-$18 per month to rental depots, depending on whether it is paid annually or monthly. Sold for $800 wholesale, MSRP is $900.

Contact

Medela, Inc. http://www.medelabreastfeedingus.com/

1.800.435.8316

Medela Symphony® (figure 143)

Figure 143. Symphony® Breast Pump, photo courtesy of Kathy Mirra.

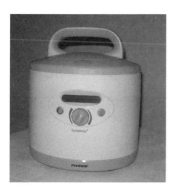

The Symphony® pump was designed to have the suction characteristics determined by a replaceable program card, similar to a video game system whose program is contained on a plug-in module. The original card (version 1.0) programmed lower suction pressures during the expression phase of pumping, and has been replaced with the more effective 2.0 card. Suction and speed are coupled according to an algorithm controlled by the program card, such that increasing the suction decreases the number of cycles per minute, with about a 40% decrease in cycles per minute when the suction is at 16 bars versus at 1 bar. This increases comfort, as mothers who are sensitive to negative pressure on their nipples (those who choose lower vacuums) are also exposed to vacuum for shorter periods of time. The vacuum does not advance a consistent amount of pressure per dial increment, some 1 unit changes increased suction 10 mmHg, others increased it 15-20 mmHg, for a range of about -40 mmHg to about -260 mmHg (in my sample Symphony 2.0), with significant pump to pump variability. The manufacturer's product specialist quotes the suction range as -50 to -250 mmHg. The suction sources for the Symphony pump are dual diaphragms, one for each breast, over which disposable flexible plastic membranes and membrane caps are placed (which are part of the personal kit for each mother). The diaphragms are replaceable, and should be replaced whenever the pump no longer produces correct suction pressures. Because the diaphragms are distal to the tubing, condensation can form in the tubes, which can lead to mold growth if not addressed. Cleaning the tubing with soapy water, and then running the pump with the tubing still attached, but the breast shields, connectors, and bottles detached will dry out the tubing. Alternatively, the tubing can be cleaned with isopropyl (rubbing) alcohol, allowing the alcohol to evaporate before reuse. Consider advising mothers of fragile babies to sanitize the tubing daily, especially when the pump is used in a hospital environment where there may be airborne pathogens that could potentially be drawn into the tubes during drying. The electric cord is detachable and replaceable. Rental stations or hospitals use a specially designed cover to discourage removal and loss of the program card or electric cord.

Symphony® Kit Assembly

Figures 144-153. Symphony® pump kit assembly, photos courtesy of Kathy Mirra.

Figure 144.

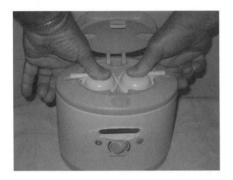

Figure 145.

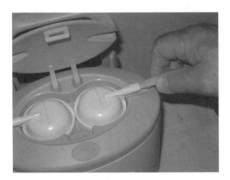

Figure 146.

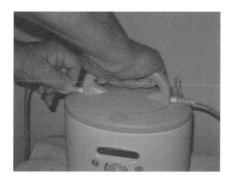

Figure 147.

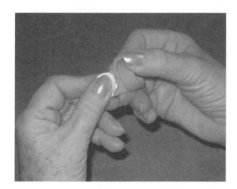

Figure 148.

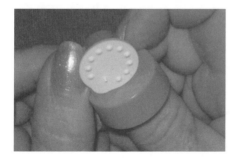

Figure 149.

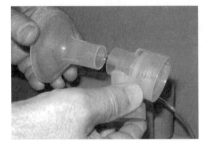

Figure 150.

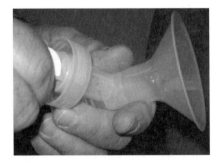

Figure 151.

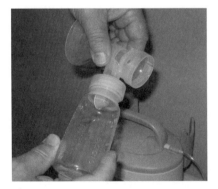

Figure 152.

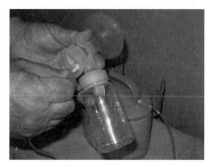

Figure 153

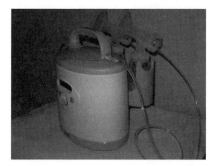

- Press the oval release button on the top of the pump to open the lid. Press the membrane caps on each membrane, being careful to direct the tube attachments outward (figure 144).

- Attach the larger, triangular cross section end of the tubing to each membrane cap (figure 145).

- Close the lid, being sure that it latches and lays flat (figure 146).

- Place the white valve into the yellow valve holder, matching up the white tab in the matching yellow slot (figure 147).

- Make certain the white valve is completely flat against the yellow valve cover (Figure 148).

- Connect the correct size breast shield to the connector (figure 149).

- Attach the valve cover and valve to the circular projection at the thread end of the connector (figure 150).

- Screw the connection container onto the connector threads (figure 151).

- Attach the transparent, circular cross section end of the tubing into the hole on the back of the connector (figure 152).

- The fully assembled kit can be placed on the holder at the rear of the pump as mother prepares to pump (figure 153).

Price

Wholesale price $950 ($190 additional for internal rechargeable batteries), Retail price is $1600 ($1800 with internal batteries). Rents for $20-$30 per month, depending on annual or monthly payment plan, and whether or not the pump has internal batteries.

Contact

Medela, Inc.   http://www.medelabreastfeedingus.com/

1.800.435.8316

Pump Trouble Shooting

Brand - Independent Problems

- The mother might have her bra cup in the way, preventing the pump kit from sealing to her breast.

- A mother with small, unusually shaped, or hypoplastic breasts may not be able to get a good seal with a standard kit, or even with a reducing insert. A softer silicone breast shield/flange like the Ameda Flexishield or Medela SoftFit breast shield may help the pump conform to her breast better.

- The motor might be worn (check pressure with a pressure gauge and a new kit).

- If the pump is accidentally plugged into a 220 volt outlet, it will usually blow the motor's safety fuse and the pump will stop functioning.

- An electric pump run for a long time (as in an engorged mother pumping for more than about 40 minutes, or a mother leaving a pump on a Sabbath timer[1] for long periods) may overheat and temporarily shut down until it cools. If this is done repeatedly, the motor may burn out. (Warn clients using a Sabbath timer to set it so the pump is on for no more than 20-30 minutes at a time.)

- Occluding the air vents during use by placing the pump on a sofa, deep pile carpet, or pillow during use may also cause it to overheat.

- Children may place small objects in any available hole in the pump, including the air port (I've found dry dog food, raisins, and coins in pumps that have been rented by families with toddlers and preschoolers).

- The tubing might have developed a pinhole, or might no longer fit tightly to the connectors.

Ameda Specific Issues

- If one side of an Ameda dual kit suddenly stops working, the problem is likely that the white valve on that side is torn or not assembled to the pump (figure 122).

- If the mother is single pumping, she may have forgotten to close off the second hole of the y connector with the attached plastic pin (figure 129).

- Elite: The piston may have gotten dirty with spilled milk, reducing the smoothness of its action. (The pistons are replaceable, see figures 112 through 116.) A worn or dirty piston will usually be noisy.

- Lact-e: The on/vacuum switch can break, making it impossible to turn the pump on/off or adjust the vacuum.

Medela Specific Issues

- The white peg with which the valve membrane attaches to the yellow valve holder may be worn, allowing air to leak through, reducing suction.

---

[1] A Sabbath timer is a device that will turn lights and appliances on and off at specified times, used by families whose religion prohibits work, including pressing buttons or using switches, during the 24 hours from Friday Sundown to Saturday Sundown. Rabbis may allow mothers to use an electric breast pump to prevent mastitis, as health concerns trump the Sabbath prohibitions in Judaic law. She may or may not be allowed to feed milk expressed on the Sabbath to her infant, depending on the Rabbi's understanding of the health consequences of replacement feeding.

- The mother may have repeatedly failed to take the valve membrane off the valve holder for cleaning, allowing it to get "glued" down with dried milk. (Washing properly restores function and hygiene!)

- The white valve membrane may be torn, distorted, or not completely flush with the valve.

- The yellow valve holder may be cracked.

- The mother may have failed to close off the second tube port if single pumping.

- The tubing may not be pushed firmly into the breast shield, or the connection may be worn.

- Classic: The white filter membrane might be wet, if so, it must be rinsed with water and allowed to air dry for 2-3 hours or dried with a blow-dryer for 10 minutes. If touched or exposed to soap, detergent, or abrasives, the filter membrane will no longer work and must be replaced.

  - The tubes may be reversed. The transparent (cylindrical) connectors get attached to the breast cup, the colored (yellow, triangular) side gets attached to the pump port.

- Symphony: The transparent diaphragms might not be properly seated, or they might be worn.

  - There might be condensation in the tubes, reducing air flow.

- Lactina: The piston cylinder might not be screwed snugly into the pump connector.

  - The rubber seal on the piston may be put on backward (the larger side goes toward the handle).

  - The cylinder, rubber seal, or vacuum regulator ring may be dirty. Medela recommends washing these parts with soap and water or vinegar and water every few uses.

  - If single pumping, the unused port connector may not be plugged tightly.

  - The tubes may be reversed. The transparent connectors get attached to the breast cup, the colored (yellow) side gets attached to the pump port.

HELPFUL TIPS

PUMPING ON ZERO FOR SORE NIPPLES.

THIS TECHNIQUE WORKS FOR PISTON AND CYLINDER ATTACHMENT FOR MEDELA LACTINA OR CLASSIC BARRIER/FILTER. OTHER PUMPS MAY ALSO BE ADJUSTABLE TO O SUCTION, WHICH IS NO SUCTION WHATSOEVER.

FOR MOTHERS WITH SO MUCH NIPPLE DAMAGE THAT THEY CANNOT BEAR THE THOUGHT OF PUMPING (EVEN TO HEAL), SHOW THEM HOW TO UNWIND THE PISTON AND CYLINDER (OR BARRIER/FILTER) TO REDUCE THE VACUUM TO O OR WHATEVER THEY CAN TOLERATE. WITH A BIT OF WATER ON THE FLANGE TO LUBRICATE THE SLIDE OF THE BREAST TISSUE ON THE FLANGE, AND KNOWING THAT THE SETTING IS AT O, NOT MINIMUM, THEY CAN TAKE CHARGE OF GRADUALLY BRINGING THE SUCTION TO NORMAL OR WHATEVER VACUUM SUCTION SETTING HELPS THEM ACHIEVE MER BY SCREWING THE PISTON OR BARRIER BACK IN PLACE. SOME ARE ABLE TO MASSAGE OR DEEP BREATHE WHILE INCREASING THE SUCTION WHILE THE MILK BEGINS TO FLOW. SUCTION IS INCREASED ONLY TO THE POINT OF NO PAIN AS GENTLE MASSAGE CAN ALSO SPEED MILK REMOVAL. SPEED ISN'T THE OBJECTIVE; IT IS COMFORTABLE MILK REMOVAL WITHOUT FURTHER NIPPLE DAMAGE. MANY MOTHERS REPORT SIGNIFICANT HEALING AND INCREASINGLY COMFORTABLE PUMPING WITHIN 48 HOURS. NIPPLES THAT DO NOT BEGIN TO HEAL WITHIN THIS PERIOD OF TIME SHOULD BE CHECKED FOR INFECTION. SOME PRACTITIONERS RECOMMEND A TINY AMOUNT OF POLYSPORIN OINTMENT AFTER PUMPINGS IF THEY SUSPECT OR WANT TO AVOID INFECTION.

JEANNE RAGO, IBCLC

Pumping/Milk Collection Accessories

Snappies®

Figure 154. Snappies® breastmilk storage containers (from left to right: 35ml, 70 ml, 13 ml)

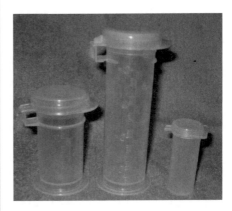

Snappies® (figure 154) is a line of sterile polypropylene (BPA free) plastic containers designed specifically for collecting human milk, ranging in size from small 13 ml containers to manually express colostrum into to 30 ml and 70 ml (2.3 oz) threaded containers that fit on a standard breast pump collection kit. The containers have an attached lid and are molded all in one piece. They are sterile by process: the manufacturing method renders them sterile on production, and the caps are closed during manufacturing to ensure an airtight, leak proof fit and maintain interior sterility. Recently, Snappies began marketing toddler snack containers and compact 2 ounce containers for transporting liquids on airplanes. (Snappies are my favorite travel containers, they have never leaked in my luggage, even on long flights, and the variety of sizes allows me to fit all my toiletries into one quart sized bag!) Bulk pricing is available for hospitals, and lactation consultants can get a sample kit to help determine which products are right for their clients by contacting Thermo Fisher Scientific customer service by email through their web form or telephone toll-free.

Snappies Breast Milk Containers
Capitol Vial Brand Products
Thermo Fisher Scientific

2039 McMillan Street
Auburn, AL 36832

800.772.8871
www.snappiescontainers.com

The two different colostrum collectors are useful for hand expression or pumping, especially when the infant is not going to be immediately fed the milk. Because Snappies have airtight covers, they are able to store milk safely. Storing colostrum in the container it was expressed into avoids loss from sticking to the sides of the container.

Lactation consultants are recommending prenatal expression of colostrum for patients who are at risk of delayed lactogenesis II (Cox, 2006), such as mothers with diabetes mellitus (Neubauer et al., 1993). Mothers are encouraged to wait until 36 weeks of pregnancy to begin expressing to minimize risk of preterm labor. The 13 ml colostrum collector is ideal for expressing drops of colostrum several times a day, refrigerating between expressions, and freezing until the birth. It is also useful for expressing colostrum in the first 24-48 hours postpartum if the newborn is unable to latch or is separated from mom, or if the baby is an inefficient feeder. Manually expressing colostrum, in addition to pumping or breastfeeding in the first days after birth, increases overall milk production. Mothers who have had insufficient milk production with previous infants could benefit from increased early stimulation. Mothers who may need to pump long term (those with preterm infants or infants with medical conditions that may negatively impact feeding ability) can also benefit from stimulating an increased milk production by increasing early demand. The 13 ml size helps to normalize typical colostrum volumes and manual expression helps prevent loss of the colostrum in pump kits. The container is narrow, but wide enough to admit a small syringe. The 13 ml container is not graduated, and has a simple hinged lid and no threads.

The 30 ml Snappies colostrum collector is threaded and designed to attach to a standard breast pump collection kit in lieu of a larger collection container. It has a gently curved bottom to help colostrum pool in the center for easy uptake in a syringe, and can be used for direct feeding of colostrum as well. The hinged lid locks open on a plastic pin to keep it clean and out of the way during use. The container has a textured area with room to write the mother's name, date, and time of expression. It is superbly balanced; the base is very stable and the container resists tipping over, even with the lid opened and locked down. This reduces the risk of losing precious colostrum during handling or transfer. The container is graduated to 35 ml, but should be filled to 30 ml for freezing to provide headroom for expansion.

Many lactation consultants recommend electric pumping after manual expression, or manual expression after electric pumping to increase milk production, especially in the first few days after birth. For mothers of preterm or ill infants, a smaller container for early pumping may help avoid disappointment that may shatter their resolve to provide milk for their babies and maintain a supply until their baby is able to breastfeed directly.

Snappies also makes a 70 ml (2.3 oz) container for pumping milk for an ill or preterm infant. They have the same lock-down hinged lid as the 30 ml size and are available in a retail package of 12 for home use ($13) or in bulk for institutions (200 for $81.) These are very useful for pumping and freezing milk, as the narrow container and smaller volume defrosts rapidly if held under cool running water or placed in a bowl of clean water. The airtight lid protects milk from contamination, evaporation, and freezer burn. The container has a stable base to prevent tipping. The container is graduated, and should be filled to 60 ml for freezing, to allow headroom for expansion. For home use, they can be washed with hot soapy water, cleaned in the top rack of a dishwasher, microwave sterilized, or boiled for 5-7 minutes after rinsing. Snappies can be reused for about 6 months. The manufacturer recommends discarding any Snappies container that becomes stained or discolored.

Use

Wash hands with soap and water or alcohol-based sanitizer. Open the lid of the Snappies container and fold it back. Hand express milk into the container, or attach to a breast pump. After use, close the container until it snaps closed, label the container as required, and refrigerate or freeze.

Price

$13 for package of 12 (retail); $81 for package of 200 (bulk for institutions)

Contact Information

Snappies Breast Milk Containers, Capitol Vial Brand Products,
Thermo Fisher Scientific, 2039 McMillan Street, Auburn, AL 36832,

1.800.772.8871

www.snappiescontainers.com

Advantages

- Sterile
- Airtight and stable to protect milk
- Attached hinged cap cannot be lost and is less vulnerable to contamination.
- Freezer safe, top rack home dishwasher safe (may melt in a commercial dishwasher)

- Multiple sizes, one for manual expression, two that can also be used with breast pumps

- Inexpensive

Disadvantages

- If not reused, create more plastic waste. (For hospitalized preterm or ill infants, re-use is discouraged in the interests of safety.)

Suggested Use

- Collect colostrum or milk for later use. The 13 ml container is also ideal for distributing small amounts of sterile liquid or gel nipple dressings, such as amorphous hydrogel or medical grade honey, to mothers.

Medela Colostrum Collection and Storage Container

Figure 155. Medela's colostrum collector has a concave bottom.

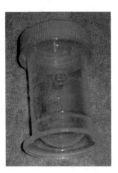

The Medela colostrum container (figure 155) is a 35 ml clarified polypropylene threaded collection bottle with a concave bottom and a screw on cap.

Use

Wash hands with soap and water or alcohol-based hand sanitizer. Open the package and remove the containers. Unscrew the lids, and carefully place on a clean surface (the inside of the packaging is ideal if it has not been contaminated). Attach the colostrum collectors to the breast pump and then secure the lids after use. Attach a label, refrigerate or freeze as required.

Price

$2 for a package of 2 (retail); $37.50 for 50 packages of 2 containers each (bulk)

Contact Information

Medela, Inc. http://www.medelabreastfeedingus.com/

1-800-435-8316

Advantages

- Sterile interior

- Concave bottom increases ease of taking milk up into a syringe, but the steep slope makes the final drops less available.

Disadvantages

- Clarified polypropylene is somewhat brittle.

- Separate cover, not airtight (Detachable covers are more vulnerable to contamination if they are not placed on a sterile surface during pumping and milk handling.)

- Can only pump 20 ml into each due to clearance needed for pump valve, but can store 35 ml.

- Expensive (a package of two retails for $2)

- Disposable (creates waste)

Suggested Use

- Use for double electric pumping during the first days postpartum. Once the packaging is open, the second container's sterility is potentially compromised, making this product less desirable for hand expression in the hospital.

Alternative for Collecting Colostrum

- An Ameda diaphragm can be interposed between the pump collection kit and the collection container. Colostrum does not adhere to the silicone material, allowing it to pool to be picked up in a syringe or poured into a storage container. It can also be used as a feeding cup to directly feed the milk to the baby. This method is ideal when the baby can be immediately fed the expressed colostrum. If the colostrum needs to be stored for later use, the diaphragm can be left inside the collection container, which can be covered by a standard threaded cap for short term storage. Figures 106-109 illustrate this technique.

HELPFUL TIPS

Susan Burger, PhD, IBCLC, finds that Pumpin' Pal's Shields can be extremely useful when mothers need to express milk frequently. Coupled with a homemade or purchased hands-free pumping bra, mothers can recline at a 45 degree angle and relax without worrying that their milk will spill out while pumping. Furthermore, these shields also seem to work well with elastic breasts. The bottom edge has a grip area to keep the breast from slipping out from underneath and the top edge has three ridges that seem to hug the breast better than the Madonna-esque cone shape of other breast shields.

Pumpin' Pal's Super Shields Plus

Figure 156. Pumpin' Pal's Super Shields Plus breast pump shield inserts

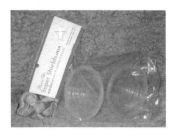

Pumpin' Pal's Super Shields Plus (figure 156) are gently tapered, ridged breast pump shield inserts to improve maternal posture and comfort during electric pumping. Molded of medical-grade polypropylene, Super Shields Plus fit into both Ameda and Medela pump kits, and provide a more steeply angled nipple tunnel to allow milk to flow into the collection container without the mother needing to lean forward. They slightly enlarge the air space of the collecting kit, which reduces the vacuum of the pump slightly. This can make pumping more comfortable for some women, and less effective for the subset that needs to use the pump's highest vacuum to empty the breast well. The bottom of the shield has raised ridges to hold the breast and discourage milk from flowing down the shield, preventing loss against the breast. Most mothers can lean back using Pumpin' Pal's Super Shields Plus without loss of milk. Super Shields can be used with hands-free pumping bras, straps (one of which is manufactured by the same company), and bustiers. Super Shields Plus come in three sizes, M, L, and XL, and are not fitted like traditional breast pump shields or flanges. They are fitted by a combination of bra size and nipple diameter. The sizing chart is available at http://www.pumpinpal.com/html/sizing_chart.htm.

Use

The Super Shield Plus nipple tunnel is pressed into the breast pump nipple tunnel with the bottom slightly rotated from the desired position and then twisted into place to secure and align.

Price

Around $13 per pair retail, wholesale prices available

Contact Information

http://www.pumpinpal.com/

1.800.466.8283

Advantages

- Improves comfort and ergonomics of breast pumps, may also improve breast drainage because the fit is more tapered
- Available in multiple sizes

Disadvantages

- May reduce peak vacuum pressure of breast pump by enlarging the nipple tunnel

Suggested Uses

- Pumpin' Pal's Super Shields are useful for mothers whose nipple-areolar junctions are injured by standard flanges because the more tapered fit puts less pressure at the base of the nipple. They improve the ergonomics of pumping, and fit a wider range of mothers than standard one size flanges. Some lactation consultants find that plugged ducts resolve more readily when a mother uses Super Shields during pumping.

Cups and Spoons

Infants who can be fed (and successfully supplemented if necessary) at breast should be fed at the breast. When the baby needs feeding and is unable to latch despite skin to skin contact and gentle enticement, alternate feeding is necessary. Alternate feeding methods are chosen to support future breastfeeding and facilitate development of feeding skills (Genna, 2008).

Fredeen (1948) prescribed cup feeding for his artificially fed patients as a way to ensure they were held for feedings. He followed these infants informally in his pediatric practice for over ten years. He compared the weight gain of 111 preterm infants fed by cup versus 59 fed by all other methods, stratified by birth weight (Fredeen, 1948). Weight gains were similar, though no statistical analysis was performed. He also tracked growth of 22 cleft lip and palate affected infants and found average growth to be 22 g per day when cup fed. Mothers were trained to hold the cup for the infant as they would hold it for themselves. Fredeen reports the feedings as sometimes loud and "gulpy," but states that there were no cases of aspiration pneumonia among his cup fed patients.

In the 1980's, Kenyan neonatologist Dr. Rachel Musoke's program to support breastfeeding in two Nairobi NICUs was featured in Breastfeeding the Low Birthweight Infant, a video produced by IBFAN Africa and UNICEF (Musoke, 1986). Universal breastfeeding was achieved at discharge and infections greatly reduced by housing mothers at the hospital, providing space for mothers to manually express milk together every 3 hours, day or night, and to cup feed their freshly expressed milk to their infants, and later to breastfeed directly (Armstrong, 1987). The video was widely distributed through UNICEF to breastfeeding supporters throughout the world, was influential in popularizing cup feeding to ease the transition to breast for preterm infants, and stimulated research on cup feeding in the U.S. and the U.K.

Howard and colleagues randomized 700 full-term breastfed infants getting supplements to cup or bottle feeding, and also examined the early (2-4 days) and late (>4 weeks) introduction of pacifiers (Howard et al., 2003). Any supplements were found to have negative effects on breastfeeding duration, as were early introduction of pacifiers. If several supplements were needed during postpartum hospitalization, cup feeding the supplements instead of bottle feeding favored longer breastfeeding duration and higher exclusivity after discharge, particularly for infants born by Cesarean section (Howard et al., 2003).

Avoiding bottles completely and supplementing gavage feeding by cup when infants were unable to breastfeed (or mother was unavailable after breastfeeding was initiated) led to 90% exclusive breastfeeding at discharge in a group of 40 preterm infants (Lang et al., 1994). Of the four "non exclusive breastfeeders" in Lang's group, two were discharged home breast and cup feeding, and two were transferred to another neonatal unit still being tube and cup fed. Lang found that when the cup was put to the infant's lips and tilted so the milk just touched the rim of the cup, infants would extend their tongue and lap the milk, bringing it into the mouth and holding it until ready to swallow. Physiologic stability was maintained, and infants frequently took more than their calculated requirement without vomiting. Figure 157 shows an infant being cup fed with a small, transparent glass mug using Lang's method, sometimes called "lip and lap".

Figure 157. Infant being cup fed by the "lip and lap" method. Note that he is being supported snugly in a sitting position, and the cup is tilted so that milk just touches his lips.

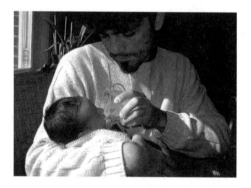

In studies where milk is poured from a cup into the infant's mouth, spillage is a significant problem. A three way crossover study in New Delhi, India, in which infants were fed by bottle, cup, and paladai (a spouted open cup used in India), feeding was faster and volumes ingested higher when feeding with the paladai; and significantly greater volumes were taken with both paladai and cup than bottle (Malhotra et al., 1999). Spillage during cup feeding was greatest for preterm infants. The poor outcomes with the cup versus the paladai in Malhotra's study may have been influenced by staff inexperience with cups. Likewise, spillage is likely to be problematic for new parents as well.

The paladai was less effective in an environment where it was the unfamiliar tool. A pilot study of paladai versus bottle to supplement preterm infants in the U.K.

found that nurses felt the paladai was more difficult for infants than bottle feeding (Aloysius & Hickson, 2007). Infants showed more stress signs during paladai feeds, and there was significantly more spillage with the paladai than the bottle. Spillage was the greatest for infants who rooted when the spout touched their lips. However, six of the fifteen infants took greater volumes of milk by paladai than bottle, four of these infants were younger than the study average gestational age. The authors comment that preterm infants may be able to safely swallow small boluses provided with appropriate pacing before coordination of sucking, swallowing, and breathing is achieved, and recommend further studies.

Cup feeding, even by the pour method, is no more stressful than bottle feeding for term infants. Physiologic stability of 98 term infants fed formula by experienced nurses via small plastic medicine cups using the pour method versus bottle did not differ significantly (Howard et al., 1999). When compared to 25 breastfeeding infants, the bottle and cup fed infants had higher respiratory and heart rates and lower oxygen saturations during and after feeding, indicating greater cardiorespiratory stress.

A crossover study of 57 preterm infants randomized to cup (lip and lap method) or bottle for their first two non-breast oral feedings found that bottle feeding resulted in higher heart rate and lower oxygen saturations (Marinelli et al., 2001), whether the infants were exposed to the cup or bottle first. Cup feeding took longer, which the authors caution should be considered more developmentally appropriate than faster, larger bolus feeding for preterm infants. A small study of preterm cup feeding (8 infants, 15 feedings in total) confirmed that feeding was slow and spillage was problematic (Dowling et al., 2002). A larger Brazilian study (78 preterm infants) supplemented by cup or bottle showed cup fed infants had fewer oxygen desaturations and twice the rate of breastfeeding at the three month follow-up among those still breastfeeding at discharge (Rocha et al., 2002). Feeding times, weight gain, volume ingested, and any breastfeeding at follow-up were similar between cup and bottle. One possible reason for the discrepancy between studies is that the infants in the Rocha et al. study were less preterm (34-36 weeks), began oral feeding at around 37 weeks, and were followed for 3 months; whereas those studied by Dowling's group had a mean gestation of 30 weeks.

An Australian study using an intent to treat model (counting infants as exposed to the method they were assigned to rather than how they were actually fed) explored the use of cups versus bottles for supplementing breastfeeding and pacifiers/dummies on breastfeeding outcomes in 303 preterm infants (Collins et al., 2004). Compliance (use of the assigned feeding method) was very poor in this study, but cup feeding was still associated with greater rates of exclusive breastfeeding at discharge (OR 1.7) and a trend toward greater prevalence of any breastfeeding at three and six months of age. Infants randomized to cup feeding had a significantly increased hospital stay (a mean of 10 days). The intent-to-treat design of this study likely underestimated the effect of cup feeding, as those who were randomized to cup feeding, but bottle

HELPFUL TIPS

fed were still identified as cup fed in data analysis. However, the intent-to-treat model identified problems with real-world implementation of cup feeding as an intervention, as failure to continue with the assigned treatment can be construed as treatment failure. There was staff resistance to cup feeding at the satellite hospitals in this study, whose personnel only had written instructions and telephone contact with the researchers as opposed to in-person training at the main sites.

Finally, an electromyographic study (Gomes et al., 2006) identified facial muscle activation during cup feeding as being more similar to breastfeeding than bottle feeding. This might provide a mechanism for easier transition to breastfeeding from cup feeding than from bottle feeding.

Specific Infant Feeding Cups

While any small cup is appropriate for use with infants, transparent or translucent cups or those with a cutout rim are particularly useful for feeding newborns.

Ameda Baby Cup

Figure 158. Ameda Baby Cup

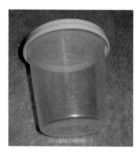

Figure 159. Ameda Baby Cups make useful containers for manual expression of milk. They are sterile and come with a cover to store milk for later feeding.

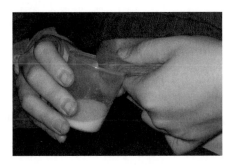

The Ameda Baby Cup (figure 158) is packed sterile in packages of 6 translucent polypropylene cups with lids. The Ameda cup holds 2 ounces (60 ml). The narrow diameter makes it easy to hold securely, yet it is wide enough for mothers to manually express milk into, as shown in figure 159. I use these cups frequently as an inexpensive, sterile container to teach mothers manual expression. They can then cover the cup and take the expressed milk home. The rim is smooth to protect the infant's mouth if the baby should move suddenly, but holds the cover in an airtight seal.

Use

Hold the infant securely against the parent's side. Place the cup to the baby's lower lip and tilt until milk just touches the rim of the cup. Allow the baby to lap the milk as in figure 157.

Price

$6.50-$7.50 per package of 6

Contact Information

Ameda Breastfeeding Products http://www.ameda.com

1.866.99.AMEDA

Advantages

- Sterile
- Airtight snap on lid
- Designed for infant feeding
- Inexpensive

Disadvantages

- Lids are no longer attached to cups in 6 pack, increasing risk of contamination once the packaging is open. When used for ill or preterm infants, either give each mother a package of six or carefully remove one cup and reseal the package to maintain cleanliness.

- The lids have been changed since the original design and the rim is now slotted (but the slot is shallow enough that it can be thoroughly cleaned). Soak in soapy water to clean the inside rim of the lid.

Suggested Use

- Use to supplement an infant who is unable to breastfeed or is obtaining insufficient milk at breast during the first few months of life.

Flexi-cup

Figure 160. Flexi-cup

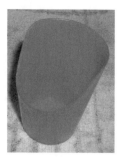

Figure 161. The feeder can easily see inside the cup, and flow is easily controlled.

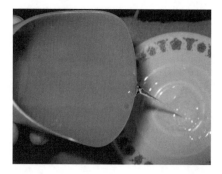

Flexi-cups (figure 160) are used by speech and occupational therapists to feed patients with limited head extension. They are flexible plastic and have a u-shaped cut out to place near the drinker's nose so that they don't need to extend their head. These cups are useful for use with infants because the feeder can use the u-shaped opening to visualize the fluid level at the infant's lip (figure 161). They come in 1 ounce capacity to the base of the U (pink) and 2 ounce (blue). The flexible plastic can be compressed to shape the rim to better fit the infant's mouth.

Use

The uncut edge of the rim is placed to the infant's lower lip. The feeder looks into the U-shaped cutout to visualize the milk level, and tilts the cup until the milk just touches the baby's lower lip. The cup can be gently squeezed to fit the baby's mouth to encourage good lip position.

Price

$8-10 per 5 cups, depending on size

Contact Information

http://www.equipmentshop.com/ProductDetail.asp?ProductID=19 and http://www.theraproducts.com/index.php?main_page=product_therapro_info&products_id=7316

Advantages

- Inexpensive
- Easy to clean
- Easy to hold
- Flow is well directed into the center of the rim (figure 161).

Disadvantages

- Easy to spill
- Not sterile

Suggested Use

- Use for cup feeding when infants require more milk than fits in smaller cups, when the infant is able to cooperate and hold still for the feeding.

Foley Cup Feeder

Figures 162-164. Foley Cup Feeder

Figure 162.   **Figure 163.**

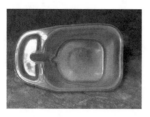   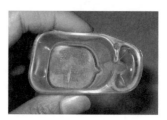

Figure 164.

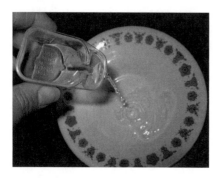

The Foley Cup Feeder is a small cup with a rim extension with a channel to control milk flow (figure 162). It was designed by parents who needed to cup feed their own newborn while their breastfeeding problems were resolved. If it is tilted slightly, milk pools in the rim extension (figure 163). If it is tilted more, a carefully controlled stream of milk flows off the center of the rim (figure 164).

Use

The infant is held securely, the Foley cup's rim extension is placed against the infant's lower lip, and the cup is held between thumb and forefinger. The cup delivers a single safe bolus of milk to the rim area.

Price

$15.00 per package of 6; $9.75 per package of 6 in lots of 50

Contact Information

Available from: http://www.foleycup.com/services.html

Advantages

- Controlled flow
- Inexpensive in bulk
- Very lightweight and easy to handle
- Autoclavable at low temperatures (250 degrees)
- Phthalate free

Disadvantages

- Small capacity
- Best for young or preterm infants or for infants who need only small amounts of supplementation. Alternatively, the small capacity limits spillage.

Suggested Use

- Ideal for young or preterm infants, very small capacity and controlled flow increase the safety of cup feeding.

Maternal Concepts® Suckle Cup™

Figure 165. Maternal Concepts® Suckle Cup™

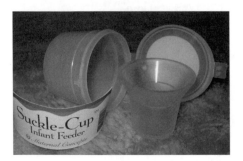

Figure 166. When tilted slightly, a slow stream of drops flows from the center of the Suckle Cup's rim.

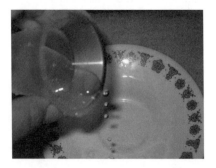

Figure 167. When tilted more, the flow increases but is still slow, well controlled, and centered on the rim.

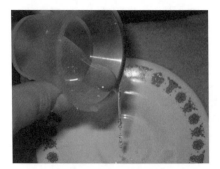

The Suckle Cup™ (figure 165) is a flexible silicone cup with an extended flared rim. It is sold in a reusable snap-top plastic container that can be used as a carrying case to keep the cup clean between uses. The graduated cup holds 20 ml to the bottom of the rim, or 30 ml if filled to mid-rim. The shape and the translucent material allow the feeder to see the fluid level during feeding. Milk does not stick to the silicone material, making the flow particularly even, and the cup is comfortable to hold. It can be used with either the lip and lap method, or milk can be poured slowly into the infant's mouth as he shows readiness for another bolus. The cup produces a very small, perfectly centered, well controlled stream of fluid when tilted, as shown in figures 166 and 167. The soft material prevents injury to the baby's lips if he should move suddenly.

Use

Fill with milk as desired, hold baby securely. Touch rim of cup to the infant's mouth and tilt until fluid just touches the lower lip. Allow the baby to drink, making sure the cup is not tilted so far that the infant is overwhelmed with flow. Wash with soap and water, rinse, air dry, and replace in storage container. Can be boiled or placed in the dishwasher for sanitization if needed.

Price

$4-$7 wholesale price depending on quantity purchased

Contact Information

Maternal Concepts http://www.maternalconcepts.com

1.800.310.5817

Advantages

- Superior flow characteristics, well designed for either cup feeding method
- Comfortable to use
- Can easily visualize fluid level
- Comes with travel container to maintain cleanliness

Disadvantages

- Easy to spill
- Relatively expensive

Suggested Use

- General cup feeding of infants, either during the newborn period or to supplement breastfeeding on an occasional basis
- Cup feeding of older babies during maternal separation

Medela Baby Cup Feeder

40 cc polypropylene cup with snap on lid, very similar to Ameda Baby cup, only smaller capacity. Most expensive simple cup.

Use

Hold to baby's lips, tilt until fluid reaches the lower lip. Allow the baby to draw the milk in with the tongue. Wash with soap and water, rinse and air dry.

Price

$12.40 for 5

Contact Information

Medela, Inc. http://www.medelabreastfeedingus.com/

1.800.435.8316

Advantages

• Cover allows cup to be transported filled.

Disadvantages

• Expensive

Suggested Use

• Cup feeding during the first few days postpartum for infants who are unable to latch or require larger amounts of supplement than can be given by spoon

Medela SoftFeeder™

Figure 168. Medela SoftFeeder™

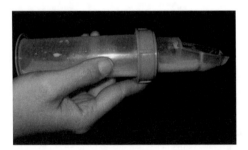

Figure 169. The small slit in the reservoir is difficult to access for cleaning.

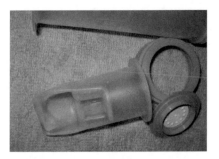

Figure 170. The feeder must be careful not to tilt the feeder too much, as milk overflows unevenly from the reservoir.

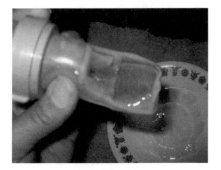

The Medela SoftFeeder™ (figure 168) is a hybrid bottle/spoon. The container is a standard 60cc bottle to which a valved soft silicone spoon-like feeding device attaches. There is a small slit on one side of the reservoir to allow flow into the silicone basin (figure 169). The basin is deep and must be tilted for the baby to access the milk. If it is tilted too far, flow off the front edge of the basin is irregular (figure 170).

Use

The baby is secured against the feeder's body. The silicone basin is placed at the infant's lip and tilted just until the infant can access the milk. The feeder repeatedly squeezes the base of the spoon chamber behind the basin to release milk. Once the basin is full of milk, it will refill without squeezing only IF no air enters the silicone reservoir. Air is kept out of the reservoir by tilting the bottle so the air bubbles rise to the rear of the container. The amount of tilt must be carefully regulated to ensure that milk does not spill from the front edge of the basin into the infant's mouth. The position of the milk must be carefully modulated so the infant is able to take respiratory breaks as needed. If the reservoir fails to refill automatically, the feeder needs to squeeze very gently to avoid liquid spraying upward into the baby's face.

Price

$16 wholesale, $32 retail

Contact Information

Medela, Inc.   http://www.medelabreastfeedingus.com/

1.800.435.8316

Advantages

- Spill resistant (Only the milk in the basin is vulnerable to spillage if the baby moves suddenly or the device is dropped.)

Disadvantages

- Expensive

- Awkward to balance in the hand, as the bottle is long and narrow. (The manufacturer warns that it may leak from the threads if used with a different bottle. Snappies containers can be used without leakage, but if a 35 ml container is used, the device does not refill automatically for long.)

- Requires squeezing at least initially, is fatiguing on the hand to use unless it is tilted sufficiently that no air enters the reservoir, in which case milk is drawn into the basin as the infant removes it.

- Does not come with a cover

- Narrow channel and position of slit makes it difficult to clean.

- Poor flow characteristics (though it is not meant to be used by the pour method)

- Bowl is deep for the lip and lap method, increasing risk of inadvertently providing large boluses.

Suggested Use

- The Softcup feeder is most useful when spillage is a significant concern. It would be better balanced and easier to handle if used with a shorter container, such as a Snappies 35 ml colostrum container.

Spoons

There are no randomized controlled trials on spoon feeding of newborns, but experience in India has demonstrated improved breastfeeding rates at discharge among preterm infants fed human milk by spoon or cup (Ramji, 2002). In an Indian comparison study, infants born by Cesarean who were provided pre-lacteal feeds by spoon were almost three times more likely to be totally breastfeeding at discharge than those initially fed by bottle (Mathur et al., 1993).

Spoons can be useful for feeding drops of expressed colostrum to newborns who are not latching to the breast to prevent hypoglycemia and excessive weight loss. Since colostrum is viscous, it can stick to containers and be lost. Expressing colostrum directly into the spoon and then allowing the infant to lick it clean helps prevent waste. Pre-wrapped, disposable plastic spoons from the mother's meal tray can be used in hospital as seen in figure 171, or well cleaned kitchen teaspoons can be used at home. Plastic coated infant spoons, plastic infant spoons, and therapeutic spoons are available and can be used to feed colostrum or milk to infants.

Figure 171. Spoon feeding colostrum from a plastic teaspoon. After the spoon feeding, the non-latching infant breastfed. Photo courtesy of Esther Grunis.

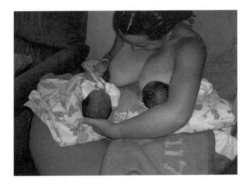

Maroon Spoon

Figure 172. Maroon spoon, smaller size

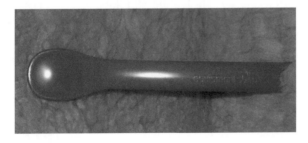

Maroon spoons (figure 172) come in small and large varieties. The maroon spoons have a shallower and narrower bowl than standard kitchen teaspoons. They are high density plastic, are easy to clean, and are durable enough to be washed in the dishwasher (they may melt if dried in the dishwasher). The shallow bowl is particularly good for feeding expressed colostrum to a small infant.

Use

Give the mother two spoons. As she expresses colostrum into one, a helper (the baby's father or other relative or health care professional) can feed colostrum to the baby with the other. The spoon should be put to the baby's lower lip and the spoon tilted until the baby can access the colostrum. The baby can either lick the colostrum off the spoon or lap it from the spoon with the lips and tongue. As the baby empties one spoon, the empty spoon can be given to the mother to refill and the spoon she was expressing into used to feed the baby. After spoon feeding several spoons, place the baby skin to skin with the mother to facilitate breastfeeding. If the mother is alone, she can alternately express into the spoon and feed her baby, or she express into a small medicine cup and feed the colostrum with a spoon.

Price

$8 per 10 spoons

Contact Information

Available from: http://www.ed-cetra.com/maroon-spoon.html

Advantages

- Inexpensive
- Easy to clean, dishwasher (wash only) safe
- Plastic is unlikely to injure infant

Disadvantages

- May melt if sterilized

Suggested Use

- Spoon feed colostrum to non-latching newborns to prevent hypoglycemia and excessive weight loss. Follow the feeding with skin to skin contact with mother to promote latching. Spoon feed milk to infants who need small amounts of supplement (larger size spoon).

Fingerfeeders

Fingerfeeding is meant to be a temporary way to nourish an infant when exclusive breastfeeding is not possible. Though several experts recommend fingerfeeding for infants who cannot latch to the breast as an alternative to bottles or cups, there is only one small study in the English language literature on finger feeding versus bottle feeding in a hospital special care nursery setting (Oddy & Glenn, 2003). Oddy & Glenn report on breastfeeding outcomes when fingerfeeding replaced bottle feeding as the final step in a hospital becoming baby friendly. Though the sample was small, a higher proportion of preterm infants were discharged breastfeeding when they were fingerfed rather than bottle fed in their mother's absence (71% versus 44%).

The biggest advantage of fingerfeeding is that it can be used to condition infants to suck more correctly. J. Joan Sheppard, PhD, CCC-SLP, and expert on suck-swallow dysphagia (swallowing difficulties in suckling infants) recommends working in function. This means that infant's oral motor skills are more amenable to correction if therapeutic techniques are used during feeding or sound production rather than at rest. Of course, infants learn to breastfeed best by practicing at the breast. When this is not possible because the infant cannot latch or cannot transfer milk even with a nursing supplementer, the mother cannot be present for every feeding, or the infant causes maternal nipple injury during sucking, fingerfeeding can be helpful. Milk flow can be allowed or interrupted depending on the infant's oral motor movements, and gentle corrective forces can be (Genna, 2008) applied by the finger to facilitate improved sucking. For example, a tongue-tied infant that uses tongue retraction and humping of the posterior tongue can be fingerfed with either gentle traction against the posterior tongue to prevent retraction or gentle corrective pressure on the posterior tongue when retraction occurs. Though no exercise can eliminate an anatomical restriction, many infants do improve their sucking skills over time with these techniques. Videos of many of these techniques are on the Health-E-Learning website in the presentation from Gold 07 entitled Finger Feeding as Oral Motor Therapy: http://www.health-e-learning.com/.

Hazelbaker™ Fingerfeeder

Figure 173. Hazelbaker™ Fingerfeeder

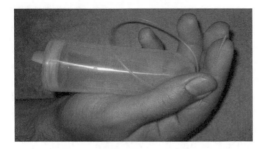

Figure 174. Placement of finger when offering the Hazelbaker™ Fingerfeeder.

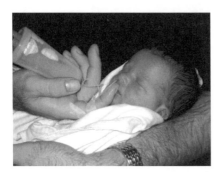

Figures 175 through 181. Hazelbaker™ Fingerfeeder assembly.

Figure 175.   Figure 176.

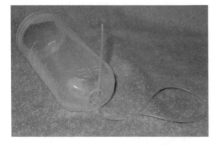 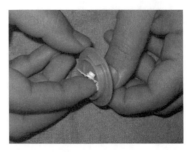

Figure 177.

Figure 178.

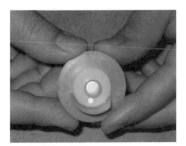

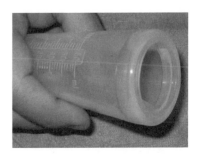

Figure 179.

Figure 180.

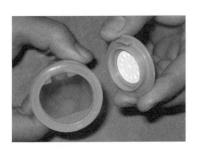

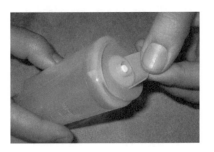

Figure 181.

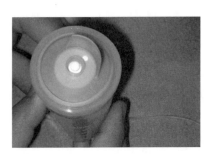

While the same devices that are used to supplement at breast can be used to fingerfeed, the Hazelbaker™ Fingerfeeder is the only device that was designed and clinically tested for use during fingerfeeding human milk and human milk substitutes. The Hazelbaker™ Fingerfeeder consists of a soft walled container that is valved at the rear and has a soft tube exiting the front. The tube is sized to provide appropriate milk flow when the baby exerts negative pressure during sucking. In contrast to manufactured nursing supplementers, which are designed to be used with a lactating breast, it is designed to be the only source of flow in the infant's mouth.

Assembly

- Crimp off the tube in the slot in the plug at the bottom of the container. Ensure that the plug is seated securely (figure 175). Margot Mann, IBCLC, likes to crimp near the front of the tube as shown in figure 175, which keeps the end of tube that will be in the baby's mouth close to the container, keeping it cleaner than if it were crimped farther back and allowed to dangle.

- Press the white valve membrane into the underside of the cap, placing the white plug through the green hole (figure 176).

- Ensure that the stem is completely through the hole and secure (figure 177).

- Fill the container. Note the container has a double wall to hold the cap in place (figure 178).

- Line up the notch in the container with the matching projection on the cap (figure 179).

- Fit the projection into the notch, then press down on the cap to seat it between the double walls (figure 180).

- Ensure the cap is fitted well into the container before use (figure 181).

Use

Place container in hand with tube exit down toward palm. Hold the tube along a finger (preferably the index or middle finger) with the thumb as in figure 173, or tape in place. Hold the baby in a comfortable feeding position, either in arms or across the lap. Encourage the baby to open the mouth wide by touching the lips with the finger (nail side toward the infant) as shown in figure 174. When the baby opens wide, encourage him to pull the finger into the mouth with the tongue (the bent finger can touch the tongue to encourage it to extend and grasp). Once the finger tip is near the junction of the hard and soft palate, release the tube from the crimp and allow the baby to transfer milk at his own pace. If bolusing is required, gently squeeze the container, but watch that the baby's respiratory capacity is not overwhelmed. Stop at any signs of stress, such as finger splaying, wide eyes, furrowed forehead, rapid breathing, or color changes.

Cleaning

Remove cover, pour out any unused milk (discard formula, human milk may sometimes be used again for a healthy, low risk infant within 5-24 hours if refrigerated). Rinse in warm soapy water, hold hand over opening and squeeze container to press soapy water through tubes, repeat with clear water. It can be autoclaved or boiled to sterilize if needed. Sterilization is more important if the device is used with manufactured milks (formula) or if the infant is preterm or hospitalized.

Price

$19 wholesale

Contact Information

Available from: Aiden and Eva, LLC, 5115 Olentangy River Road, Columbus, Ohio 43235

1.614.451.1154

Advantages

- Designed for fingerfeeding, clinical research conducted during development
- Created by an IBCLC
- Infant controls milk flow
- Easy to use, one handed operation

Disadvantages

- Relatively expensive, but the device is reusable indefinitely, avoid applying traction to the tubing where it attaches to the container

Suggested Use

- When infants are unable to breastfeed and require stimulation to the tongue to help correct sucking, fingerfeeding is a helpful way to feed.

Alternatives

- A syringe and tube, curved tip syringe, or a Lact-Aid or SNS can be used for fingerfeeding as well.

When using an active flow device (one where the parent presses a syringe to deliver milk), flow should be provided at the correct time in the suck cycle (when the posterior tongue pulls down). Flow should be interrupted when the baby stops for a respiratory pause (about 3-5 seconds every 10-30 sucks), and the feeder should be alert for stress cues and alterations to the infant's respiratory pattern that indicate the flow is too fast. Chele Marmet, IBCLC, recommends using a curved tip syringe (periodontal syringe) for fingerfeeding to allow very controlled milk flow as shown in figure 182. Careful control of flow is vital for infants with cardiorespiratory problems or infants who are sucking incorrectly and need help learning what movements produce milk flow at the breast without causing maternal pain. Many parents find a syringe and tube easier to handle and sufficiently accurate. The syringe and tube allows more freedom in positioning the infant for fingerfeeding than a curved tip syringe does as illustrated by figure 183.

Figure 182. Fingerfeeding with curved tip syringe

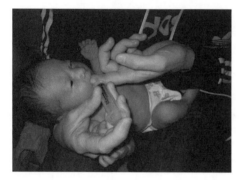

Figure 183. Hand position for fingerfeeding with the curved tip syringe. The tip of the syringe is pressed against the feeder's finger to protect the infant's mouth.

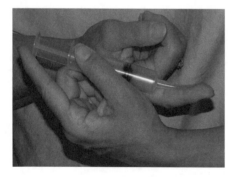

Figure 184. Fingerfeeding with a syringe and tube may allow a more comfortable hand position, but still gives good flow control.

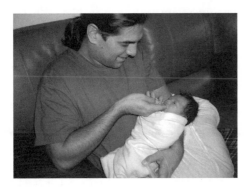

Figure 185. Fingerfeeding in a prone position with mild head extension, using the SNS and its narrowest tubing, helped this infant with Laryngomalacia practice coordinating swallowing and breathing so she could transition to breastfeeding.

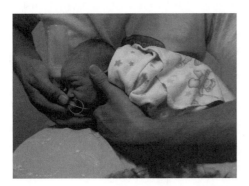

Figure 186. The Hazelbaker Fingerfeeder can be used as a supplementer when particularly high flow is needed.

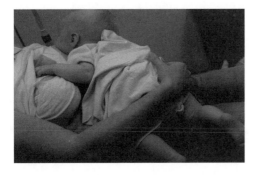

Devices that require vacuum to release milk, such as nursing supplementers and the Lact-Aid, can also be used for fingerfeeding, but these devices are not designed to provide the only flow in the infant's mouth and should be used judiciously. For infants with cardiorespiratory anomalies, this slower flow may be ideal. The infant in figure 185 had a respiratory anomaly which made coordinating swallowing and breathing initially problematic. A day of fingerfeeding with the SNS providing very slow flow allowed her to improve her coordination and breastfeed.

For undernourished infants or preterm babies, the effort of feeding using a device intended for supplementation at the breast may be too great and may compound their problems. Certainly, supplementer devices can be used on the finger before breastfeeding to help organize an infant's sucking, or the remainder of the supplement can be fingerfed to the infant after breastfeeding to avoid wasting human milk. Conversely, if the mother has already invested in a Hazelbaker Fingerfeeder and needs to give the baby added flow at the breast, the fingerfeeder can be used as a supplementer with the understanding that the flow will be more rapid than devices that are designed for supplementation at breast. A rapid flow can be useful to help transition a reluctant infant to breast. Figure 186 illustrates an infant at breast for the first time after frenotomy using the Hazelbaker Fingerfeeder as a supplementer.

Sometimes multiple fingerfeeding devices can be used serially to help an infant develop their sucking skills. Starting with a syringe and tube and moving to a more difficult device can help a baby work toward better intraoral vacuum production, which can correlate with better milk transfer at the breast.

Conclusion

New products are constantly being developed and marketed to fill real and perceived needs of breastfeeding families. One of the roles of the lactation consultant is to investigate the features and shortcomings of new devices and advise clients on which tools may be useful in specific situations. Far too many families buy items that are unsuitable for their needs, wasting resources and sometimes even endangering breastfeeding. Once resources are squandered on an unhelpful device, fewer dollars are left for appropriate lactation care. How many of us have had to try to convince a mother struggling to initiate milk production that she would be better served by renting a hospital grade pump when she has already spent hundreds of dollars on an ineffective one? If mothers look to lactation consultants to provide unbiased, scientific information about breastfeeding products, family finances, the IBCLC profession, and breastfeeding outcomes all benefit. I hope this book provided useful information to make clinical judgments about breastfeeding tools.

References

Alexander, J. M., Grant, A. M., & Campbell, M. J. (1992). Randomised controlled trial of breast shells and Hoffman's exercises for inverted and non-protractile nipples. *BMJ, 304,* 1030-1032.

Aloysius, A. & Hickson, M. (2007). Evaluation of paladai cup feeding in breast-fed preterm infants compared with bottle feeding. *Early Human Development, 83,* 619-621.

Armstrong, H. (1987). Breastfeeding low birthweight babies: advances in Kenya. *Journal of Human Lactation, 3,* 34-37.

Arsenault, G. (1997). Using a disposable syringe to treat inverted nipples. *Canadian Family Physician, 43,* 1517-1518.

Ashton, R. & Leppard, B. (2004). *Differential diagnosis in dermatology.* Abingdon: Radcliffe.

Auerbach, K.G. (1990). The effect of nipple shields on maternal milk volume. *Journal of Obstetric, Gynecologic, and Neonatal Nursing, 19,* 419-427.

Benakappa, A. (2002). A new Lact-aid technique. *Indian Pediatrics, 39,* 1169.

Benbow, M. & Vardy-White, C. (2004). Study into the effectiveness of Mothermates. *British Journal of Midwifery, 12,* 244-248.

Bodley, V. & Powers, D. (1996). Long-term nipple shield use--a positive perspective. *Journal of Human Lactation, 12,* 301-304.

Borucki, L.C. (2005). Breastfeeding mothers' experiences using a supplemental feeding tube device: finding an alternative. *Journal of Human Lactation, 21,* 429-438.

Brent, N., Rudy, S. J., Redd, B., Rudy, T. E., & Roth, L. A. (1998). Sore nipples in breast-feeding women: a clinical trial of wound dressings vs conventional care. *Archives of Pediatrics and Adolescent Medicine, 152,* 1077-1082.

Broad, F.E. (1975). Further studies on the effects of infant feeding on speech quality. *New Zealand Medical Journal, 82,* 373-376.

Broad, F.E. & Duganzich, D.M. (1983). The effects of infant feeding, birth order, occupation and socio-economic status on speech in six-year-old children. *New Zealand Medical Journal, 96,* 483-486.

Cable, B. & Davis, J. (1998). Hydrogel dressings not to be used on infected tissue. *Journal of Human Lactation, 14,* 205.

Cable, B., Stewart, M., & Davis, J. (1997). Nipple wound care: a new approach to an old problem. *Journal of Human Lactation, 13,* 313-318.

Cadwell, K., Turner-Maffei, C., Blair, A., Brimdyr, K., & Maja, M.Z. (2004). Pain reduction and treatment of sore nipples in nursing mothers. *The Journal of Perinatal Education, 13,* 29-35.

Capuco, A.V., Ellis, S.E., Hale, S.A., Long, E., Erdman, R.A., Zhao, X., et al. (2003). Lactation persistency: insights from mammary cell proliferation studies. *Journal of Animal Science, 81 Suppl 3*, 18-31.

Carrascoza, K.C., Possobon, R.F., Tomita, L.M., & Moraes, A.B. (2006). Consequences of bottle-feeding to the oral facial development of initially breastfed children. *Journal d Pediatria (Rio J.), 82*, 395-397.

Chertok, I.R., Schneider, J., & Blackburn, S. (2006). A pilot study of maternal and term infant outcomes associated with ultrathin nipple shield use. *Journal of Obstetric, Gynecologic, and Neonatal Nursing, 35*, 265-272.

Clum, D. & Primomo, J. (1996). Use of a silicone nipple shield with premature infants. *Journal of Human Lactation, 12*, 287-290.

Collins, C.T., Ryan, P., Crowther, C.A., McPhee, A.J., Paterson, S., & Hiller, J.E. (2004). Effect of bottles, cups, and dummies on breast feeding in preterm infants: a randomised controlled trial. *BMJ, 329*, 193-198.

Cooper, R.A., Molan, P.C., Krishnamoorthy, L., & Harding, K.G. (2001). Manuka honey used to heal a recalcitrant surgical wound. *European Journal of Clinical Microbiology & Infectious Diseases, 20*, 758-759.

Cotterman, K.J. (2004). Reverse pressure softening: a simple tool to prepare areola for easier latching during engorgement. *Journal of Human Lactation, 20*, 227-237.

Cox, N. & Hinkle, R. (2002). Infant botulism. *American Family Physician, 65*, 1388-1392.

Cox, S.G. (2006). Expressing and storing colostrum antenatally for use in the newborn period. *Breastfeeding Review, 14*, 11-16.

Delatte, S. J., Evans, J., Hebra, A., Adamson, W., Othersen, H. B., & Tagge, E. P. (2001). Effectiveness of beta-glucan collagen for treatment of partial-thickness burns in children. *Journal of Pediatric Surgery, 36*, 113-118.

Densmore, L. & Pflueger, S. M. (2008). Using interphase fluorescence in situ hybridization (I-FISH) to detect the transfer of infant cells during breastfeeding. *Journal of Human Lactation, 24*, 401-405.

Dewey, K.G., Nommsen-Rivers, L.A., Heinig, M.J., & Cohen, R.J. (2003). Risk factors for suboptimal infant breastfeeding behavior, delayed onset of lactation, and excess neonatal weight loss. *Pediatrics, 112*, 607-619.

Dodd, V. & Chalmers, C. (2003). Comparing the use of hydrogel dressings to lanolin ointment with lactating mothers. *Journal of Obstetric, Gynecologic, and Neonatal Nursing, 32*, 486-494.

Dowling, D.A., Meier, P.P., DiFiore, J.M., Blatz, M., & Martin, R.J. (2002). Cup-feeding for preterm infants: mechanics and safety. *Journal of Human Lactation, 18*, 13-20.

Efem, S. E. (1988). Clinical observations on the wound healing properties of honey. *The British Journal of Surgery, 75*, 679-681.

Egnell, E. (1956). The mechanisms of different methods of emptying the female breast. *Journal of the Swedish Medical Association, 40*.

Eisenbud, D., Hunter, H., Kessler, L., & Zulkowski, K. (2003). Hydrogel wound dressings: where do we stand in 2003? *Ostomy/Wound Management, 49*, 52-57.

Falanga, V. & Iwamoto, S. 2008. Wound repair: Mechanisms and practical considerations" (Ch. 249). In Wolff, K., Goldsmith, L.A., Katz, S.I., Gilchrest, B., Paller, A.S., & Leffell, D.J. (Eds.) *Fitzpatrick's dermatology in general medicine*, 7th Ed. McGraw Hill. http://www.accessmedicine.com/content.aspx?aID=3006805.

Fredeen, R. C. (1948). Cup feeding of newborn infants. *Pediatrics, 2,* 544-548.

Geddes, D.T. & McClellan H.L. (2007, May) *Sucking difficulties of breastfed babies: what the research shows.* Paper presented at the College of Lactation Consultants of Western Australia, Seeking Suckling Success: Recent Research – Proven Practice, Freemantle, Western Australia.

Genna, C.W. (2008). *Supporting sucking skills in breastfeeding infants.* Sudbury, Mass: Jones and Bartlett Publishers.

Gerosa, F., Baldani-Guerra, B., Lyakh, L.A., Batoni, G., Esin, S., Winkler-Pickett, R.T., et al. (2008). Differential regulation of interleukin 12 and interleukin 23 production in human dendritic cells. *The Journal of Experimental Medicine, 205,* 1447-1461.

Glover, R. (2005). *Follow me mum: The key to successful breastfeeding* (Revised ed.). [Video recording]. Perth, Western Australia: Tapestry Films.

Glover, R. & Wiessinger, D. (2008). The infant-maternal breastfeeding conversation: Helping when they lose the thread. In C.W. Genna (Ed.), *Supporting sucking skills in breastfeeding infants* (1st ed., pp. 97-129). Sudbury, MA: Jones and Bartlett Publishers.

Gomes, C.F., Trezza, E.M., Murade, E.C., & Padovani, C.R. (2006). Surface electromyography of facial muscles during natural and artificial feeding of infants. *Journal of Pediatrics (Rio J), 82,* 103-109.

Guóth-Gumberger, M. (2006). Parent-info: Breastfeeding with the supplementary nursing system. [Pamphlet]. Hannover, Germany: Elwin Staude Verlag, Deutsche Hebammenzeitschrift.

Guóth-Gumberger, M. (2008, October). Making a supplemental feeding tube device work for a baby with a cleft palate. Presented at VELB/ILCA Conference *A World Wide View on Breastfeeding* (proceedings pp. 94-95), Vienna, Austria.

Hale, T.W. (2008). *Medications and mothers' milk 2008.* (13th ed.) Amarillo, TX: Hale Pub., L.P.

Henriques, A., Jackson, S., Cooper, R., & Burton, N. (2006). Free radical production and quenching in honeys with wound healing potential. *The Journal of Antimicrobial Chemotherapy, 58,* 773-777.

Herzog-Isler, C. (2008, October). Born at home - with a cleft palate - a case history. Presented at VELB/ILCA Conference *A World Wide View on Breastfeeding* (proceedings pp. 93), Vienna, Austria.

Hill, P.D. & Aldag, J.C. (2005). Milk volume on day 4 and income predictive of lactation adequacy at 6 weeks of mothers of nonnursing preterm infants. *The Journal of Perinatal & Neonatal Nursing, 19,* 273-282.

Hill, P.D., Aldag, J.C., & Chatterton, R.T. (1999). Effects of pumping style on milk production in mothers of non-nursing preterm infants. *Journal of Human Lactation, 15,* 209-216.

Hoover, K.L., Barbalinardo, L.H., & Platia, M.P. (2002). Delayed lactogenesis II secondary to gestational ovarian theca lutein cysts in two normal singleton pregnancies. *Journal of Human Lactation, 18*, 264-268.

Howard, C.R., de Blieck, E.A., ten Hoopen, C.B., Howard, F.M., Lanphear, B.P., & Lawrence, R.A. (1999). Physiologic stability of newborns during cup- and bottle-feeding. *Pediatrics, 104*, 1204-1207.

Howard, C.R., Howard, F.M., Lanphear, B., Eberly, S., deBlieck, E.A., Oakes, D., et al. (2003). Randomized clinical trial of pacifier use and bottle-feeding or cupfeeding and their effect on breastfeeding. *Pediatrics, 111*, 511-518.

Huggins, K.E., Petok, E.S., & Mireles, O. (2000). Markers of lactation insufficiency: A study of 34 mothers. In K.G. Auerbach (Ed.). *Clinical issues in human lactation* (pp. 25-35). Sudbury, MA: Jones and Bartlett.

Ikewaki, N., Fujii, N., Onaka, T., Ikewaki, S., & Inoko, H. (2007). Immunological actions of Sophy beta-glucan (beta-1,3-1,6 glucan), currently available commercially as a health food supplement. *Microbiology & Immunology, 51*, 861-873.

Johnson, D.W., Van, E.C., Mudge, D.W., Wiggins, K.J., Armstrong, K., Hawley, C.M., et al. (2005). Randomized, controlled trial of topical exit-site application of honey (Medihoney) versus mupirocin for the prevention of catheter-associated infections in hemodialysis patients. *Journal of the American Society of Nephrology, 16*, 1456-1462.

Jones, E., Dimmock, P.W., & Spencer, S.A. (2001). A randomised controlled trial to compare methods of milk expression after preterm delivery. *Archives of Disease in Childhood: Fetal and Neonatal Edition, 85*, F91-F95.

Kent, J.C., Mitoulas, L.R., Cregan, M.D., Geddes, D.L.M., Doherty, D.A., & Hartmann, P.E. (2008). Importance of vacuum for breastmilk expression. *Breastfeeding Medicine, 3(1)*, 11-19.

Kesaree, N., Banapurmath, C.R., Banapurmath, S., & Shamanur, K. (1993). Treatment of inverted nipples using a disposable syringe. *Journal of Human Lactation, 9*, 27-29.

Kougias, P., Wei, D., Rice, P. J., Ensley, H. E., Kalbfleisch, J., Williams, D. L. et al. (2001). Normal Human Fibroblasts Express Pattern Recognition Receptors for Fungal (1{right-arrow}3)-{beta}-D-Glucans. *Infection and Immunity, 69*, 3933-3938.

Labiner-Wolfe, J., Fein, S.B., & Shealy, K.R. (2008). Infant formula-handling education and safety. *Pediatrics, 122 Suppl 2*, S85-S90.

Lang, S., Lawrence, C.J., & Orme, R.L. (1994). Cup feeding: an alternative method of infant feeding. *Archives of Diseases in Childhood, 71*, 365-369.

Lau, C. & Schanler, R.J. (1996). Oral motor function in the neonate. *Clinics in Perinatology, 23*, 161-178.

Lavigne, L.M., Albina, J.E., & Reichner, J.S. (2006). Beta-glucan is a fungal determinant for adhesion-dependent human neutrophil functions. *Journal of Immunology, 177*, 8667-8675.

LeBlanc, B.W., Albina, J.E., & Reichner, J.S. (2006). The effect of PGG-{beta}-glucan on neutrophil chemotaxis in vivo. *Journal of Leukocyte Biology, 79*, 667-675.

Leite-Cavalcanti, A., Medeiros-Bezerra, P.K., & Moura, C. (2007). Breast-feeding, bottle-feeding, sucking habits and malocclusion in Brazilian preschool children. *Revista de Salud Pública, 9,* 194-204.

Lerrer, B., Zinger-Yosovich, K.D., Avrahami, B., & Gilboa-Garber, N. (2007). Honey and royal jelly, like human milk, abrogate lectin-dependent infection-preceding Pseudomonas aeruginosa adhesion. *The ISME Journal, 1,* 149-155.

Lescano de Ferrer, A. & Varela de Villalba, T.B. (2006). Effect of the suction-swallowing action on orofacial development and growth. *Revista de la Facultad de Ciencias Médicas (Cordoba, Argentina) 63,* 33-37.

Livingstone, V. & Stringer, L.J. (1999). The treatment of Staphylococcus aureus infected sore nipples: a randomized comparative study. *Journal of Human Lactation, 15,* 241-246.

Luhm, J., Langenkamp, U., Hensel, J., Frohn, C., Brand, J.M., Hennig, H., et al. (2006). Beta-(1-->3)-D-glucan modulates DNA binding of nuclear factors kappaB, AT and IL-6 leading to an anti-inflammatory shift of the IL-1beta/IL-1 receptor antagonist ratio. *BMC Immunology, 7,* 5.

Lusby, P.E., Coombes, A.L., & Wilkinson, J.M. (2005). Bactericidal activity of different honeys against pathogenic bacteria. *Archives of Medical Research, 36,* 464-467.

MAIN Trial Collaborative Group. (1994). Preparing for breast feeding: treatment of inverted and non-protractile nipples in pregnancy. The MAIN Trial Collaborative Group. *Midwifery, 10,* 200-214.

Malhotra, N., Vishwambaran, L., Sundaram, K.R., & Narayanan, I. (1999). A controlled trial of alternative methods of oral feeding in neonates. *Early Human Development, 54,* 29-38.

Marinelli, K.A., Burke, G.S., & Dodd, V.L. (2001). A comparison of the safety of cupfeedings and bottlefeedings in premature infants whose mothers intend to breastfeed. *Journal of Perinatology., 21,* 350-355.

Mathur, G.P., Pandey, P.K., Mathur, S., Sharma, S., Agnihotri, M., Bhalla, M. et al. (1993). Breastfeeding in babies delivered by cesarean section. *Indian Pediatrics, 30,* 1285-1290.

McGeorge, D.D. (1994). The "Niplette": an instrument for the non-surgical correction of inverted nipples. *British Journal of Plastic Surgery, 47,* 46-49.

Meier, P.P., Brown, L.P., Hurst, N.M., Spatz, D.L., Engstrom, J.L., Borucki, L.C., et al. (2000). Nipple shields for preterm infants: effect on milk transfer and duration of breastfeeding. *Journal of Human Lactation, 16,* 106-114.

Molan, P.C. & Allen, K.L. (1996). The effect of gamma-irradiation on the antibacterial activity of honey. *The Journal of Pharmacy & Pharmacology, 48,* 1206-1209.

Musoke, R. N. (1986). Breastfeeding the Low Birthweight Infant. [Video recording]. Nairobi, Kenya: IBFAN/UNICEF.

Neubauer, S.H., Ferris, A.M., Chase, C.G., Fanelli, J., Thompson, C.A., Lammi-Keefe, C.J. et al. (1993). Delayed lactogenesis in women with insulin-dependent diabetes mellitus. *American Journal of Clinical Nutrition, 58,* 54-60.

Newman, J. (1997). Caution regarding nipple shields. *Journal of Human Lactation, 13,* 12-13.

Newman, J. (2005). Handout #4. Is My Baby Getting Enough? Revised January 2005. http://www.thebirthden.com/Newman.html. Accessed November 23, 2008.

Nyqvist, K.H. (2008). Early attainment of breastfeeding competence in very preterm infants. *Acta Paediatrica, 97,* 776-781.

Oddy, W.H. & Glenn, K. (2003). Implementing the Baby Friendly Hospital Initiative: the role of finger feeding. *Breastfeeding Review, 11,* 5-10.

Ogbuanu, I.U., Karmaus, W., Arshad, S.H., Kurukulaaratchy, R.J., & Ewart, S. (2009). Effect of breastfeeding duration on lung function at age 10 years: a prospective birth cohort study. *Thorax, 64(1),* 62-66.

Ohyama, M., Watabe, H., Hayasaka, Y., Saito, K., & Mizuguchi, H. (2007). Which is more effective, manual or electric expression in the first 48 hours after delivery in a setting of mother-infant separation? A Preliminary Report. *Breastfeeding Medicine 2(3),* 179.

Okan, D., Woo, K., Ayello, E.A., & Sibbald, G. (2007). The role of moisture balance in wound healing. *Advances in Skin & Wound Care, 20,* 39-53.

Ozcan, M. & Kahveci, R. (1995). The 'Niplette' for the non-surgical correction of inverted nipples. *British Journal of Plastic Surgery, 48,* 115.

Palmer, B. (1998). The influence of breastfeeding on the development of the oral cavity: a commentary. *Journal of Human Lactation, 14,* 93-98.

Pohl, L. (2003, October). An engineer looks at breastfeeding tools. Paper presented at NYLCA Advanced Practice Conference, New York, NY.

Porter, J. & Schach, B. (2004). Treating sore, possibly infected nipples. *Journal of Human Lactation, 20,* 221-222.

Powers, D. & Tapia, V.B. (2004). Women's experiences using a nipple shield. *Journal of Human Lactation, 20,* 327-334.

Ramji, S. (2002). Enteral feeding of low birth weight infants. *Indian Journal of Pediatrics, 69,* 401-404.

Rocha, N.M., Martinez, F.E., & Jorge, S.M. (2002). Cup or bottle for preterm infants: effects on oxygen saturation, weight gain, and breastfeeding. *Journal of Human Lactation, 18,* 132-138.

Simon, A., Sofka, K., Wiszniewsky, G., Blaser, G., Bode, U., & Fleischhack, G. (2006). Wound care with antibacterial honey (Medihoney) in pediatric hematology-oncology. *Supportive Care in Cancer, 14,* 91-97.

Slater, M. (2008). Does moist wound healing influence the rate of infection? *British Journal of Nursing (BJN), 17,* S4-15.

Smith, L. (2008). Coach Smith's rules for breastfeeding helpers. Retrieved February 17, 2008 from http://www.bflrc.com.

Suharyono & Paul, M. (1997). Breastfeeding practices in Indonesia. *Zhonghua Min Guo Xiao Er Ke Yi Xue Hui Za Zhi, 38,* 338-344.

Tanzi, M.G. & Gabay, M.P. (2002). Association between honey consumption and infant botulism. *Pharmacotherapy, 22,* 1479-1483.

Terrill, P.J. & Stapleton, M.J. (1991). The inverted nipple: to cut the ducts or not? *British Journal of Plastic Surgery, 44,* 372-377.

Tonks, A., Cooper, R.A., Price, A.J., Molan, P.C., & Jones, K.P. (2001). Stimulation of TNF-alpha release in monocytes by honey. *Cytokine, 14,* 240-242.

Tonks, A.J., Cooper, R.A., Jones, K.P., Blair, S., Parton, J., & Tonks, A. (2003). Honey stimulates inflammatory cytokine production from monocytes. *Cytokine, 21,* 242-247.

Tonks, A.J., Dudley, E., Porter, N.G., Parton, J., Brazier, J., Smith, E.L., et al. (2007). A 5.8-kDa component of manuka honey stimulates immune cells via TLR4. *Journal of Leukocyte Biology, 82,* 1147-1155.

Tsikitis, V.L., Albina, J.E., & Reichner, J.S. (2004). Beta-glucan affects leukocyte navigation in a complex chemotactic gradient. *Surgery, 136,* 384-389.

Vardi, A., Barzilay, Z., Linder, N., Cohen, H.A., Paret, G., & Barzilai, A. (1998). Local application of honey for treatment of neonatal postoperative wound infection. *Acta Paediatrica, 87,* 429-432.

Visavadia, B.G., Honeysett, J., & Danford, M.H. (2008). Manuka honey dressing: An effective treatment for chronic wound infections. *The British Journal of Oral & Maxillofacial Surgery, 46,* 55-56.

Walker, M. (2005). Breast pumps and other technologies. In J. Riordan (Ed.), *Breastfeeding and Human Lactation* (3rd ed.) (pp. 323-365). Sudbury, Mass: Jones and Bartlett.

Wei, D., Zhang, L., Williams, D.L., & Browder, I.W. (2002). Glucan stimulates human dermal fibroblast collagen biosynthesis through a nuclear factor-1 dependent mechanism. *Wound Repair & Regeneration, 10,* 161-168.

Weichert, C.E. (1980). Prolactin cycling and the management of breast-feeding failure. *Advances in Pediatrics, 27,* 391-407.

Wiessinger, D. (1998). A breastfeeding teaching tool using a sandwich analogy for latch-on. *Journal of Human Lactation, 14,* 51-56.

Wiessinger, D. (2000). My baby just doesn't get it. Retrieved February 17, 2008 from http://www.wiessinger.baka.com/bfing/trouble/babyget.html.

Wilson-Clay, B. (1996). Clinical use of silicone nipple shields. *Journal of Human Lactation, 12,* 279-285.

Wilson-Clay, B. & Hoover, K. (2005). *The breastfeeding atlas.* (3rd ed.). Manchaca, TX: LactNews Press.

Woolridge, M.W., Baum, J.D., & Drewett, R.F. (1980). Effect of a traditional and of a new nipple shield on sucking patterns and milk flow. *Early Human Development, 4,* 357-364.

W

About the Author

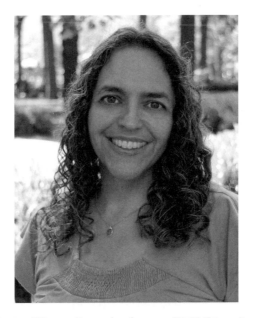

Catherine Watson Genna has been an IBCLC in private practice in NYC since 1992. She has a special interest in the anatomical, genetic and neurological influences on infant sucking skills, and writes and speaks on these topics. She is co-researcher in a study utilizing ultrasound to examine tongue movements during breastfeeding in infants with ankyloglossia and other sucking problems. Her clinical photographs have been published in both lay and scholarly venues. *Selecting and Using Breastfeeding Tools* (Hale Publishing, 2009) is her second book, joining *Supporting Sucking Skills in Breastfeeding Infants* (Jones and Bartlett Publishers, 2007).

Ordering Information

Hale Publishing, L.P.

1712 N. Forest Street

Amarillo, Texas, USA 79106

❖

8:00 am To 5:00 pm CST

❖

Call » 806.376.9900

Sales » 800.378.1317

Fax » 806.376.9901

❖

Online Web Orders

www.ibreastfeeding.com

❖